CMSRN Exam Prep 2023-2024

Complete Review + 450 Questions and Detailed Answer Explanations for the Medical-Surgical Registered Nurse Certification Exam (Study Guide + 3 Full-Length Exams)

Table of Contents

Chapter 1: Medical-Surgical Nursing Certification

Introduction

Welcome to your CMSRN (Certified Medical-Surgical Registered Nurse) study guide. This guide is written to help you prepare for the CMSRN exam and achieve certification as a medical-surgical nurse. The exam is administered by the Medical-Surgical Nursing Certification Board (MSNCB) and tests your knowledge and skills in the care of adult medical-surgical patients.

This study guide includes a literature review and 450 questions, with explanatory answers covering the topics included in the 2023 CMSRN Exam Blueprint/Test Specifications.

Each question tests your knowledge and understanding of the material, and the explanations provided will help you understand the concepts and principles behind the correct answers. By studying the questions and explanations in this guide, you will be better prepared to pass the CMSRN exam.

Keep in mind that the guide is not a substitute for hands-on experience and continuing education in medical-surgical nursing. The guide is intended to supplement your knowledge and understanding of the concepts and principles essential to the care of adult medical-surgical patients.

We hope this guide will be a valuable resource as you prepare for the CMSRN exam.

Good luck on your journey to certification!

About the CMSRN Certification

The CMSRN certification is a professional certification program offered by the MSNCB, which recognizes the knowledge and skills of medical-surgical nurses who provide care to adult patients with acute and chronic conditions.

Obtaining CMSRN certification is an important milestone in a medical-surgical nurse's career, as it demonstrates a commitment to professional development and excellence in practice. This certification is recognized by employers and other health care professionals as a measure of competence and expertise. It is a requirement for many advanced practice nursing roles and leadership positions within the medical-surgical nursing field. Holding CMSRN certification can also bring professional benefits, such as increased job opportunities, higher pay and increased credibility.

The exam covers a wide range of topics, including patient assessment, diagnosis and treatment, medication management and patient education. The CMSRN certification is valid for a period of five years. After five years, nurses who wish to maintain their certification must complete the recertification process.

Eligibility

To be eligible for the CMSRN certification exam, you must meet the following requirements:

- Have a current, unrestricted registered nurse (RN) license in the United States and its territories, or Canada
- Have completed a minimum of 2,000 hours of medical-surgical nursing practice in the past three years
- Have a minimum of two years of experience as an RN in a medical-surgical setting

In addition to these requirements, you must also agree to adhere to the MSNCB Code of Ethics.

Application Instructions

Once you have determined that you meet the eligibility requirements, you can complete the application process by following these steps:

1. Visit the amsn.org website and apply.
2. To ensure that you fulfill the eligibility conditions, the MSNCB will evaluate the application.

3. You will receive an email including the exam receipt after finishing the application registration.
4. Once your request to schedule your exam has been granted, you will receive your Authorization to Test (ATT) in a second email. The exam must be taken within 90 days of receiving your ATT.

CMSRN Exam Details

The CMSRN exam is a computer-based exam that consists of 150 multiple-choice questions, of which 125 are scored, and 25 are unscored pretest questions. The exam is three hours in length, and you are allowed to take breaks during the exam as needed.

Before the CMSRN exam begins, you will be given a 10-minute tutorial to familiarize yourself with the exam format and instructions. Once the exam is completed, you will be given a five-minute post-test survey. These time periods are not included in the three-hour testing time.

The CMSRN exam is accessible at physical testing locations or remotely through Prometric, all of which adhere to security and administration regulations.

In-Person Exam Information

- Arrive 30 minutes before your appointment to allow for check in.
- At the test location, lockers will be available for you to store your personal belongings, such as handbags, backpacks and bulky coats. Personal belongings are your responsibility; Prometric is not liable for them. Prometric advises leaving them at a different, more secure location of your choosing.
- Once your identification has been confirmed, the testing facility will be made available to you. You will be seated randomly.
- A proctor will actively monitor candidates using an observation window, audio and video recording and other means.
- The exam clock will continue to run even if you take a break. Before continuing the exam, you may have to go through the check-in process again.

Remote Proctor

- Before setting up a Prometric remote proctored exam, you should perform a systems readiness check, read the FAQ and familiarize yourself with common technical problems.
- The Google Chrome browser and a laptop or desktop computer are required to take the test.

- Your computer must include functioning speakers, a microphone and a webcam that can be moved around to assess the testing location for security issues.
- For security purposes, your space, jewelry and glasses will be inspected. You must take the test in a room with a closed door.
- During the exam, no one else may be in the room with you or come in. The exam will be stopped if this happens, and you will not be able to retake it without submitting a new application and payment.
- Unplanned breaks are allowed, but you cannot leave the room and the exam clock will still be running. You will have to go through the check-in procedure again when you return and connect with a proctor.

Restrictions

1. No phone, camera, book, notes, programmable electronic device, or any kind of recording device is allowed in the CMSRN exam.
2. No jewelry is allowed other than wedding or engagement jewelry.
3. No eating, drinking or smoking is allowed while taking the exam.
4. Copying or leaking exam content is prohibited by state law and security protocol. Either of these could invalidate exam results and result in legal action.

Fee Information

Fees can change without notice at any time. To be sure you get the most updated information, go to msncb.org.

Regular candidates must pay an application fee of $394; AMSN members pay $267.

Before submitting the certification application, register at amsn.org to receive the member pricing. All application prices include a $79 processing fee, which is not refundable.

Chapter 2: Patient/Care Management

Patient Safety

There are several key concepts and best practices that medical-surgical nurses should be familiar with in order to promote patient safety and pass the CMSRN exam.

1. **Infection control** – Understand the types of microorganisms that can cause infections, as well as the transmission pathways and preventive measures that can be used to reduce the risk of infection. This includes hand hygiene, the use of personal protective equipment (PPE) and proper cleaning and sterilization of equipment.
2. **Medication administration** – Understand the different routes of medication administration, as well as the proper dosage. Nurses should also be familiar with the potential side effects, interactions of medications and the importance of monitoring patients for these effects.
3. **Patient identification** – Ensure that patients are correctly identified before administering medication, performing procedures or making other important decisions about their care, which can be done through a variety of methods, such as using name bands, checking identification cards or having patients state their name and date of birth.
4. **Risk assessment and fall prevention** – Falls are a common event in the hospital setting and can result in serious injury. Nurses need to be familiar with risk factors that increase the likelihood of falls and also preventive measures that can be taken to minimize these risks.
5. **Communication** – Clearly and compassionately convey information to patients and their families, as well as collaborate effectively with other members of the health care team. This includes verbal communication and written communication, such as charting and documenting patient information. Nurses should also be familiar with The Joint Commission's National Patient Safety Goals (NPSGs) and how they relate to their practice.

Table 1. Fall Prevention Guidelines for Nurses

Fall Prevention Guidelines for Nurses	Description
Assess fall risk	Assess each patient's fall risk upon admission and reevaluate the risk regularly throughout their stay. Factors to consider include age, mobility, cognitive function, medications and history of falls.
Implement fall prevention strategies	Use of bed alarms, bed rails and nonslip mats, as well as assistive devices, such as canes or walkers.
Use assistive devices	Encourage patients to use assistive devices when walking and moving around. Ensure that the devices are the proper fit and in good working condition.
Monitor medications	Monitor patients' medications, particularly those that may affect balance or cause drowsiness. Report any concerns to the physician and make appropriate adjustments to the medication regimen.
Keep the environment safe	Ensure that the patient's room and surrounding areas are free of tripping hazards and that any necessary equipment is within easy reach. Keep floors dry and clean.
Promote mobility	Encourage patients to move and ambulate as much as possible to maintain strength and balance.
Educate patients and families	Educate patients and their families about fall prevention strategies and the importance of reporting any falls or near misses.
Collaborate with the interdisciplinary team	Collaborate with the interdisciplinary team, including physical therapy and occupational therapy, to develop an individualized fall prevention plan for each patient.

Nursing Process

The five steps of the nursing process are assessment, diagnosis, planning, implementation and evaluation.

Assessment – The first step in the nursing process is gathering and organizing data about the patient. This particularly involves conducting interviews, reviewing the patient's medical history and observing and measuring vital signs. A physical examination is also performed to assess the patient's overall health and identify any potential issues. This information is then used to form a comprehensive understanding of the patient's current health status.

Diagnosis – The second step is identifying any actual or potential health problems based on the information gathered during the assessment step. It consists of formulating a diagnosis statement that includes the problem, the cause of the problem and related symptoms, which are then organized using a standardized taxonomy to make it easier to plan and implement care.

Planning – In this phase, the care team establishes goals and objectives for the patient's care, which includes setting priorities based on the patient's condition and needs, developing a care plan and selecting appropriate interventions. The care plan is then documented to ensure that all team members are aware of the patient's individualized care plan.

Implementation – The fourth step is putting the care plan into action. This includes providing the patient with the appropriate interventions and treatments, as well as monitoring the patient's progress and response to care.

Evaluation – The final step is evaluating the effectiveness of the care provided and making any necessary adjustments, which consists of assessing whether the patient has achieved the desired outcomes and goals, and if not, reevaluating the care plan and making any necessary changes to ensure the patient receives the best possible care.

Patient Safety Protocols

The NPSGs are a set of guidelines established by The Joint Commission, an independent, nonprofit organization that accredits and certifies health care organizations and programs in the United States. These goals are intended to improve the safety and quality of care provided by health care organizations and reduce the risk of errors and adverse events.

The NPSGs cover a wide range of topics, including communication, infection control, medication management and patient rights. They are updated annually, and organizations must demonstrate compliance in order to maintain their accreditation.

The National Patient Safety Goals

The NPSGs for a health care organization include several specific guidelines that must be met to demonstrate compliance. Some of the key NPSGs are discussed in the following table.

Table 2. National Patient Safety Goals

Improve the accuracy of patient identification

- Medical-surgical nurses are responsible for verifying the identity of patients before administering any treatment or medication by using two patient identifiers, such as the patient's name and date of birth, every time care is provided.

Enhance communication among caregivers

- Medical-surgical nurses often work with a team of health care professionals, including physicians, physical therapists and social workers. Clear communication among all team members is crucial for ensuring that patients receive the best possible care.

Improve the safety of using medications

- Medication errors are a common cause of patient harm. Medical-surgical nurses are responsible for administering medication correctly, monitoring patients for potential side effects and reporting any errors or adverse reactions.

Reduce the risk of infections associated with medical care

- Medical-surgical nurses should follow infection-control guidelines, including hand hygiene, use of PPE, environmental cleaning, identifying and isolating infected patients, educating the patient and the family and being aware of facility-specific policies and guidelines.

Protect every patient from potential harm from falls

- To protect every patient from potential harm from falls, medical-surgical nurses should follow guidelines and best practices, including conducting fall-risk assessments, implementing fall prevention strategies, managing medication, identifying and addressing environmental hazards, educating patients and their families and being aware of facility-specific policies and guidelines.

Identify, resolve and prevent adverse events

- Medical-surgical nurses should be aware of the signs and symptoms of adverse events and report any incidents to their supervisor. Once an adverse event has been reported, a thorough investigation should be conducted to determine the root cause of the event and any contributing factors.
- Based on the findings of the investigation, corrective actions should be implemented.

Prevent health care–related pressure ulcers

- Assess patients for their risk of developing pressure ulcers upon admission and then continue monitoring for this risk regularly throughout their care.

Keep in mind that these are just some examples and that there are many other NPSGs in addition to those listed here. You can find them on The Joint Commission website at www.jointcommission.org, covering a wide range of areas related to patient safety and quality of care.

Risk Factors

There are various types of risks that can affect patient safety and quality of care, which can be classified into different categories, as discussed in the table below.

Table 3. Risk Factors and Examples

Risks	
Pharmacological risks	Risks associated with medications, such as adverse drug reactions, medication errors and drug interactions. Examples of pharmacological risks include allergic reactions to medication, incorrect dosage and incorrect timing.
Environmental risks	Risks associated with the physical environment, such as falls, infections and exposure to hazardous materials. Examples of environmental risks include slippery floors, poor lighting and poor ventilation.
Equipment risks	Risks associated with medical equipment, such as malfunction, improper use and lack of maintenance. Examples of equipment risks include malfunctioning equipment, equipment not being properly sterilized or cleaned, and equipment not being properly stored.
Demographic risks	Risks associated with patient demographics, such as age, gender and underlying medical conditions. Examples of demographic risks include older adults having a higher risk of falls and patients with underlying medical conditions, such as diabetes, having a higher risk of infection.
Human factor risks	Risks associated with human error, such as communication errors, fatigue and distraction. Examples of human factor risks include miscommunication between members of the health care team; nurses working long

	shifts, leading to fatigue and burnout; and distractions leading to medication errors.
Psychological risks	Risks associated with a patient's mental health, such as depression, anxiety and stress. Examples of psychological risks include patients with depression not adhering to their treatment plan and patients with anxiety not cooperating with the health care team.
Cultural risks	Risks associated with cultural and linguistic differences, such as misunderstandings and the lack of an understanding of the patient's beliefs and values.
Economic risks	Risks associated with patients' financial resources, such as lack of access to health care, lack of insurance or difficulty paying for treatment. Examples of economic risks include patients not getting the necessary treatment because they cannot afford it and patients not being able to pay for the treatment they receive.
Legal and ethical risks	Risks related to legal and ethical issues, such as informed consent, patient autonomy and end-of-life care. Examples of legal and ethical risks include patients not being fully informed about their treatment options, patients not being allowed to make decisions about their care and patients not receiving appropriate end-of-life care.

Risk Assessment Tools

To identify and mitigate these risks, nurses can use a variety of risk assessment tools, such as preoperative assessment, checklists, time-out procedures, anesthesia evaluation, postoperative assessment, incident reporting and continuous quality improvement.

Preoperative assessment is a tool to identify any potential risks before surgery. This includes evaluating the patient's medical history and physical condition and reviewing laboratory results.

Checklists can be used to ensure that all necessary steps are taken before, during and after surgery to prevent errors and complications.

Time-out is a standardized procedure that is performed before the start of surgery to confirm the correct patient, procedure and surgical site.

Anesthesia evaluation examines the patient's response to anesthesia and monitors vital signs to ensure that the patient is stable throughout the procedure.

Postoperative assessment is essential to monitor the patient's vital signs, pain levels and wound healing after surgery to identify and address any potential complications.

Incident reporting is a tool to identify and report any adverse events, near misses or unsafe practices during the surgery so that the data can be analyzed and recurrences prevented.

Continuous quality improvement (CQI) is an ongoing process that involves regularly evaluating and improving the surgical process based on the data collected from incident reporting.

Patient Safety Culture

Patient safety culture contains the shared values, beliefs, behaviors and practices within an organization that contribute to the prevention of errors and adverse events in health care.

The World Health Organization (WHO) recognizes the importance of a strong safety culture in the health care setting and has identified it as a key factor in ensuring patient safety. The WHO has listed safety culture as one of the 10 human factors relevant to patient safety.

A strong patient safety culture includes several key elements, such as:

Near-miss reporting – Encouraging the reporting of near misses and incidents, regardless of their severity, allows for the identification of underlying problems and systems issues and the development of strategies to address them.

Just culture – A just culture is one in which individuals are not punished for honest mistakes but are held accountable for reckless or intentional actions. This allows for a culture of open communication where staff feels safe to report errors without fear of retaliation, which improves the quality of care and helps prevent future incidents.

Speak up – (**S** – Speak Up; **P** – Pay Attention; **E** – Educate Yourself; **A** – Advocate; **K** – Know About Your New Medicine; **U** – Use a Quality Health Care Organization; **P** – Participate in All Decisions About Your Care).

Speak Up is an initiative The Joint Commission developed to encourage patients to be informed and involved in their care, ask questions and voice concerns about their treatment.

By providing patients with the knowledge and skills they need to communicate effectively with their health care providers, the initiative aims to empower them to take an active role in preventing errors and ensuring their own safety. Encouraging staff and patients to speak up when they notice something that does not seem right is vital to building a culture of safety. Giving employees and patients a voice enables them to be active participants in identifying and resolving issues before they lead to errors or adverse events.

High-accountability organizations – High-accountability organizations ensure that all employees understand their roles and responsibilities in ensuring patient safety and are held accountable for their actions. In this way, everyone in the organization takes ownership of safety and is responsible for creating and maintaining a culture of safety.

Care Bundles

Care bundles are a set of evidence-based practices that, when implemented together, have been shown to improve patient outcomes. They typically consist of a checklist of specific actions that should be taken for a particular medical condition or procedure, as well as an algorithm to guide decision-making. Care bundles are used in many areas of medicine, including critical care, surgery and primary care. Many different types of care bundles have been developed for different medical conditions and procedures. Some examples are:

Surgical care improvement project (SCIP) bundles – These bundles are designed to improve the quality and safety of care for patients undergoing surgery and include guidelines for preoperative care, intraoperative care and postoperative care.

Ventilator-associated pneumonia bundles – These are designed to prevent ventilator-associated pneumonia (VAP), a common complication of mechanical ventilation, and include guidelines for preventing infections, such as hand hygiene, oral care and stress ulcer prophylaxis.

Sepsis bundles – These are designed to improve the identification and management of sepsis, a life-threatening complication of infection. They include guidelines for early identification, appropriate antibiotic therapy and supportive care.

Central line–associated bloodstream infection bundles – These are designed to prevent central line–associated bloodstream infections (CLABSI), a common complication of central venous catheters. They include guidelines for hand hygiene, the use of sterile techniques and appropriate care of the catheter site.

Pneumonia bundles – These are designed to improve the quality of care for patients with pneumonia and include guidelines for antibiotics, oxygen therapy and other treatments.

Stroke care bundle – These are designed to improve care for stroke patients and can include guidelines for early identification, administration of clot-busting medications and rehabilitation.

The items on the checklists can vary depending on the specific care bundle, but they generally include specific steps that should be taken before, during and after the procedure or treatment.

For example, a checklist for preventing VAP might include:

1. Head of the bed elevation
2. Oral care
3. Stress ulcer prophylaxis
4. Sedation vacation

A checklist for a stroke care bundle could include:

1. Recognition and activation of emergency medical services
2. Rapid assessment and diagnosis
3. Use of thrombolytic therapy (clot-busting medication) if appropriate
4. Early initiation of rehabilitation

An algorithm is a set of step-by-step instructions that are used to guide decision-making and are often used in conjunction with checklists to provide a structured approach to care and ensure that all necessary steps are taken. An example of a pain management algorithm would involve:

1. Assessing the patient's pain level.
2. Identifying the cause of the pain.
3. Selecting an appropriate pain management technique.
4. Administering the chosen treatment.
5. Monitoring the patient's response to the treatment.
6. Adjusting the treatment as needed.

Algorithms like these provide a structured approach to care, which is often reviewed and updated regularly to reflect changes in best practices and evidence-based care. They can also be used as a quality metric in health care organizations.

Patient Safety Assessment and Reporting

Patient safety assessment is the process of identifying and evaluating potential hazards that could harm patients in a health care setting and implementing measures to prevent these hazards. This is a process that involves monitoring and analyzing data related to patient safety, as well as conducting on-site assessments of health care facilities to identify areas of risk.

There are several steps in the process of patient safety assessment:

Identification of hazards – Reviewing patient data, monitoring incident reports and conducting on-site assessments to identify areas of risk.

Evaluation of risks – Analyzing the potential impact of identified hazards on patient safety and the likelihood of their occurrence.

Control and prevention – Implementing interventions to prevent identified hazards. This can include staff training, protocol development and process improvement initiatives.

Monitoring and evaluation – Ongoing monitoring and evaluation of the effectiveness of interventions and making adjustments as necessary.

Communication and education – Sharing information about identified hazards and interventions with staff, patients and other stakeholders to promote a culture of safety and encourage participation in safety efforts.

Patient Safety Reporting

Patient safety reporting is the process of identifying and reporting incidents or conditions that have the potential to harm patients or negatively impact the quality of care provided. The goal of patient safety reporting is to identify problems and issues related to patient safety as soon as possible so that appropriate actions can be taken to prevent harm. Patient safety reporting can be done in a variety of ways, including:

Incident reporting – Submitting reports of specific incidents or adverse events that have occurred, such as medication errors or falls.

Root cause analysis – Investigating the underlying causes of incidents or adverse events and identifying ways to prevent them from happening again in the future.

Near-miss reporting – Reporting incidents that did not cause harm but had the potential to do so.

Patient complaints – Patient complaints can also be considered a form of reporting, which can help identify issues related to patient safety and quality of care.

When it comes to patient safety reporting, **abuse, human trafficking and social determinants of health** should be considered potential hazards that need immediate attention.

A medical-surgical nurse who suspects a patient is a victim of abuse should follow the proper reporting protocol established by the health care facility.

The first step would be to document the suspected abuse in the patient's medical record, including any observations or statements made by the patient; this documentation should be as detailed and specific as possible, including descriptions of any injuries or other observable evidence of abuse.

The nurse should also inform the supervisor or designated abuse reporting contact immediately, who will then proceed with mandatory reporting to the appropriate authorities, such as police or child protective services.

Furthermore, the nurse should provide emotional support and information to the patient about the available resources and options, such as safe housing and counseling services, if the abuse is related to domestic violence.

In many regions, health care providers are mandatory reporters, meaning that by law, they must report any suspicion of abuse to the authorities. Thus, the nurse should also be familiar with the reporting laws and regulations in the area and ensure compliance with them.

Social determinants of health (SDOH) refer to the social and economic factors that can affect a person's health. These can include things like income, education and access to health care.

In terms of reporting and addressing SDOH, health care providers may use a variety of methods to identify and understand the social factors that are impacting a patient's health, such as:

- Assessing patients for SDOH during clinical encounters by using standardized screening tools or asking specific questions related to a patient's living and working conditions, education or access to food or transportation
- Collecting data and analyzing it to identify patterns and trends related to SDOH among a specific population or within a specific community
- Collaborating with community-based organizations or other partners to develop interventions that address the SDOH identified through screening and analysis

Health care providers can take many actions to address SDOH, such as:

- Making appropriate referrals to community resources, such as affordable housing or food assistance programs, when a patient is found to be facing social barriers that are affecting their health
- Coordinating care with other service providers and community organizations to ensure that patients are getting the support they need to address the social factors affecting their health
- Advocating for policy and system changes that will help address the underlying social factors that are negatively impacting health, such as lack of affordable housing, unemployment or inadequate transportation options

Human trafficking – Health care providers may be among the first to come into contact with a victim of human trafficking, and as such, they have an important role in identifying and reporting suspected cases. To identify potential victims of human trafficking, health care providers can look for signs such as:

- Physical signs of abuse, neglect or torture
- Fearful or anxious behavior, especially when interacting with law enforcement or immigration authorities
- Lack of identification documents or possession of false documents
- Presence of tattoos or branding that may indicate the person is a victim of trafficking
- Evidence of being controlled or coerced, such as having someone else speak for them or being accompanied by a controlling person
- Unexplained or inconsistent details in the patient's story

If a health care provider suspects that a patient is a victim of human trafficking, they should immediately inform their supervisor or designated trafficking reporting contact and report it to the appropriate authorities, such as police or federal agencies dedicated to combating human trafficking.

A health care provider should provide emotional support and information to the patient about the available resources and options, such as safe housing, legal and social services and counseling. Maintaining patient confidentiality and avoiding putting them in danger by informing the suspected traffickers about their report or the patient's location is a must.

Risk Assessment Methods

Risk assessment is a key part of patient safety that helps ensure that patients receive safe, high-quality care and that adverse events are minimized. Medical-surgical nurses can use several risk assessment methods, which are explained in the table below.

Table 4. Risk Assessment Methods and Proper Examples

	Definition	**Example**
Root cause analysis (RCA)	It is a process that helps identify the underlying cause of an incident or problem. It is used to identify the symptoms, gather data, analyze the data and identify the root cause(s) of the problem. By identifying the root cause of a problem, RCA helps identify areas for improvement and develop strategies to prevent similar incidents from occurring in the future.	A patient in the medical-surgical unit develops deep vein thrombosis (DVT) after surgery. An RCA is conducted to identify the root cause of the DVT. The RCA team finds that the patient was not properly assessed for DVT risk before surgery and was not given appropriate prophylaxis during surgery. The RCA team recommends that all patients be properly assessed for DVT risk before surgery and that appropriate prophylaxis be given to high-risk patients.
Failure mode and effects analysis (FMEA)	FMEA is a process that helps identify potential failure modes in a process or system and assess the potential consequences of those failure	An FMEA is conducted on the process of administering medication. The FMEA team identifies potential failure modes, such as incorrect medication administration, incorrect dosage and

	modes. By identifying potential failure modes and assessing their potential consequences, FMEA helps identify and prioritize potential risks and develop and implement control plans to mitigate them.	incorrect timing. They also assess the potential consequences, such as adverse drug reactions, medication errors and patient harm. The FMEA team recommends implementing a double-check system for medication administration and providing additional education for nurses on medication administration.
Safety rounds	Safety rounds involve physically walking through the workplace and looking for potential hazards or unsafe conditions.	The safety round team identifies hazards, such as a wet floor in the bathroom, a broken bed rail and a missing handrail in the hallway, then reports these hazards to the appropriate staff, who take steps to address them.
Safety huddles	Safety huddles involve a brief, daily meeting to discuss safety issues and identify and address any concerns. This method helps ensure that hazards and unsafe conditions are identified and addressed promptly.	The safety huddle team discusses a recent adverse event that occurred in the unit, such as a patient falling out of bed. The team discusses the event and identifies potential ways to prevent similar events from occurring in the future, such as placing bed alarms on high-risk patients.

Infection Prevention

Universal and Transmission-Based Precautions

OSHA Guidelines for Infection Prevention

OSHA, the Occupational Safety and Health Administration, is a federal agency that is dedicated to ensuring the safety and well-being of employees in the workplace. It sets guidelines and regulations to protect workers from potential hazards and injuries, including exposure to infectious materials.

Employers are required to implement standard policies and procedures to protect their employees and provide them with appropriate PPE, such as gloves, gowns, masks and eye protection. Proper disposal of sharps is mandated by OSHA, as well as safe work practices, such as effective hand hygiene.

Precautions

When a patient is admitted with or develops an infection that poses a risk to others, infection-control measures must be implemented.

The Centers for Disease Control and Prevention (CDC) has established guidelines with two levels of precautions: standard precautions, which are applied to all patients in hospitals and health care facilities, and transmission-based precautions, which are specific to certain diseases. The purpose of these precautions is to prevent the spread of infectious organisms from patients to health care providers, other patients and people outside the hospital. Standard precautions apply to blood, bodily fluids, secretions, excretions, nonintact skin and mucous membranes and reduce the risk of transmission of microorganisms in hospitals. They should be applied to all patients regardless of their diagnosis or infection status.

Transmission-based precautions are used for patients known or suspected to be infected with highly transmissible or epidemiologically important pathogens that require additional measures to interrupt transmission and prevent infection. These include airborne, droplet and contact precautions.

Airborne precautions are used if the organism can cause infection over long distances when suspended in the air (TB, rubeola).

Droplet precautions are used to minimize contact with pathogens that are spread through the air at close contact and that affect the respiratory system or mucous membranes (influenza, pertussis).

Contact precautions are an essential measure in preventing the spread of pathogens that are acquired through direct or indirect contact, particularly multidrug-resistant organisms (MDROs), such as MRSA and VRE. These precautions are implemented to reduce the risk of transmission from patients to health care providers and other patients. Transmission-based precautions may be combined for diseases that have multiple routes of transmission.

Infection-Control Practices and Standards

Table 5. CDC Infection-Control Recommendations

Infection-Control Measures	Description
Hand sanitation	Perform hand sanitation using soap and water or alcohol-based sanitizer after coming into contact with potentially contaminated surfaces, before and after treating patients and when entering and exiting a patient's room.
Protective gear	Wear appropriate PPE, such as gloves, gowns, masks, goggles or face shields, when performing procedures that have a risk of exposure to bodily fluids or contaminated surfaces.
Equipment decontamination	Use proper decontamination techniques, such as cleaning and disinfecting, to prevent the spread of germs on frequently touched surfaces and medical equipment.
Air filtration	Ensure that the air ventilation system in patient rooms and treatment areas is equipped with high-efficiency particulate air (HEPA) filters that can capture airborne pathogens.
Isolation protocol	Implement isolation protocols for patients with contagious illnesses to prevent the spread of infection to other patients or health care workers.
Waste management	Properly dispose of medical waste and contaminated materials to prevent the spread of infection.
Patient education	Educate patients on infection prevention measures, such as proper hand hygiene and respiratory etiquette.
Employee health screening	Regularly screen employees for symptoms of infectious diseases and require them to stay home if they are sick to prevent the spread of infection in the workplace.
Emergency preparedness	Develop and regularly update emergency preparedness plans for outbreaks of infectious diseases.

Evidence-Based Practice for Infection Control and Prevention Procedures

The WHO provides guidelines and recommendations for a range of topics, including hand hygiene, environmental cleaning and the appropriate use of PPE. The WHO also guides the prevention and control of specific types of infections, such as surgical site infections and health care–associated infections (HAIs) caused by multidrug-resistant organisms.

Surgical site infections (SSIs) are a common type of HAI that can occur following surgical procedures. SSIs can lead to increased patient morbidity, prolonged hospital stays and increased health care costs. The WHO recommends several evidence-based strategies to prevent SSIs. These involve:

- **Proper hand hygiene** – Health care workers should perform hand hygiene with soap and water or an alcohol-based hand sanitizer before and after each patient contact and before and after performing invasive procedures.
- **Appropriate surgical attire** – Health care workers should wear clean, sterile gloves, a surgical gown and a mask or face shield during surgical procedures.
- **Prophylactic antibiotics** – When appropriate, prophylactic antibiotics should be administered to patients before surgical procedures to reduce the risk of SSIs.
- **Proper wound management** – The surgical wound should be closed in a way that minimizes the risk of infection and promotes healing.
- **Proper patient positioning** – To minimize pressure on the surgical wound, patients should be positioned in a way that promotes good circulation and reduces the risk of injury.
- **Proper environmental cleaning and disinfection** – The environment in which the surgical procedure is performed should be cleaned and properly disinfected to minimize the risk of infection.

HAIs caused by MDROs are a growing concern in health care settings worldwide. MDROs are strains of bacteria, viruses, fungi and parasites that are resistant to multiple types of antibiotics and are difficult to treat.

The WHO recommends several strategies to prevent the spread of MDROs:

Infection-control measures – Proper hand hygiene, use of PPE and appropriate cleaning and disinfection of health care environments are essential in preventing the spread of MDROs.

Active surveillance – Regular monitoring of patients, staff and the environment for the presence of MDROs is important to identify and isolate infected individuals and to implement appropriate infection-control measures.

Antimicrobial stewardship – Programs that promote the appropriate use of antibiotics, including the use of narrow-spectrum antibiotics and the avoidance of unnecessary antibiotic use, can reduce the development and spread of MDROs.

National action plans – Governments should develop national action plans to combat the spread of MDROs in health care settings, including guidelines for infection control, antimicrobial stewardship and monitoring and reporting of infections.

The WHO also recommends other measures to prevent the spread of MDROs in health care settings, including:

- **Patient placement** – Patients infected or colonized with MDROs should be placed in private rooms or rooms with other patients infected or colonized with the same organism to minimize the risk of transmission.
- **Contact precautions** – Patients infected or colonized with MDROs should be placed on contact precautions, which include using gloves and gowns when entering the patient's room and using dedicated equipment and supplies for the patient.
- **Airborne precautions** – Patients infected or colonized with MDROs that can be transmitted through the air, such as tuberculosis or COVID-19, should be placed on airborne precautions, which include the use of masks and eye protection and negative air pressure rooms when available.
- **Education and training** – Regular training and education of health care workers on the proper use of PPE, hand hygiene and infection-control measures are essential to prevent the spread of MDROs.

Antimicrobial Stewardship

Antimicrobial stewardship is a comprehensive approach that aims to optimize the use of antibiotics and other antimicrobial agents to reduce the emergence and spread of antibiotic-resistant organisms. The central goal of this program is to ensure that patients receive the most appropriate therapy in terms of drug choice, dosage, duration and route of administration. By promoting the rational use of antimicrobials, stewardship programs strive to improve patient outcomes, reduce health care costs and decrease the burden of antibiotic resistance.

There are several key components of an antimicrobial stewardship program:

- **Surveillance** – Regular monitoring of antibiotic use, resistance patterns and patient outcomes is necessary to identify areas where improvements in antibiotic use can be made. This includes tracking the emergence and spread of antibiotic-resistant organisms, such as methicillin-resistant Staphylococcus aureus (MRSA), multidrug-resistant Escherichia coli and others.

- **Education** – Regular training and education of health care workers, patients and the general public about the appropriate use of antibiotics and the risks of antibiotic resistance is essential. This includes educating health care workers on the appropriate use of common antibiotics, such as penicillins, tetracyclines, macrolides, fluoroquinolones and cephalosporins, which can cause resistance when used inappropriately.

- **Guidelines and protocols** – The development and implementation of guidelines and protocols for the appropriate use of antibiotics can help ensure that antibiotics are prescribed only when necessary and that the most appropriate drug is selected. This includes ensuring that narrow-spectrum antibiotics are used whenever possible and that broad-spectrum antibiotics are used only when necessary.

- **Feedback and audit** – Regular feedback and audit of antibiotic prescribing practices can help identify areas where improvements can be made and track progress over time. This includes monitoring prescribing trends, tracking resistance patterns and evaluating the effectiveness of interventions.

- **Interventions** – Interventions, such as formulary restriction, de-escalation of therapy, switching to a narrower-spectrum antibiotic and optimizing dosing and duration of therapy, are key strategies of antimicrobial stewardship.

- **Supportive culture** – Creating a culture in which health care workers feel comfortable questioning antibiotic prescriptions and discussing alternatives with prescribing physicians is essential. This includes fostering an environment where health care workers feel comfortable discussing the risks and benefits of different treatment options with their patients and colleagues.

Medication Management

Safe Medication Administration Practices

Medication administration requires significant attention to detail to prevent errors and adverse reactions, and one of the most critical stages of this process is the transition point, such as the ordering and preparing phase, where errors are more likely to occur.

Parenteral medications, including those administered via IV or SC, are considered high-alert medications due to the potential for significant harm when used in error. To ensure the safe administration of medication, health care professionals should be well-versed in the following:

- Safe dosage range for each medication they administer
- Clearly labeling and storing in their original containers medications that are prepared away from the bedside
- Referring to lists of high-alert medications and avoiding using error-prone abbreviations or look-alike drugs and symbols
- Verifying the medication and dosage before administering it to the patients, never assuming an ordered medication is correct

Errors can also occur if the incorrect equipment is used to prepare the medication or if errors occur in the preparation, administration or post-assessment of the patient. These errors can lead to complications, such as nerve or tissue damage, medication being absorbed too quickly or too slowly, administering medication to the wrong location, pain, bleeding or even a sterile abscess.

Adverse reactions can still happen despite all precautions taken to ensure safe medication delivery. Any health product might cause an unfavorable reaction, which can range from a mild side effect like a skin rash to a significant and potentially fatal event like a heart attack or liver damage. It is crucial to be aware of potential drug side effects and report them as soon as they arise, because these reactions can happen minutes or even years after exposure to the product.

Patient Medication Education

The process of patient medication education entails informing patients about their medication, including its use, dose, administration, possible side effects and any necessary precautions. Patients should be given this information in an understandable and straightforward manner and their questions and concerns should be taken into consideration. Patients should be given written materials to refer to later during the teaching process, such as medication guides or pamphlets. Make certain that patients are aware of how to take their medications correctly, including the appropriate quantity and frequency, as well as how to store them. Additionally, patients should be made aware of any possible side effects of their drugs and what to do in such cases. They should be advised to notify their physician right away if they have any negative reactions or side effects. The precautions patients must take while taking the drugs, such as avoiding particular foods or activities, should also be explained to them.

Health care professionals should periodically check in with patients to make sure they understand and are correctly following the prescription regimen. Medication education for patients should be a continuous effort. This can be accomplished at routine check-ups or subsequent appointments.

Polypharmacy

The polypharmacy problem—using several prescriptions or possibly needless or unsuitable medications—is getting more and more common as the health care sector develops. This may occur when a patient uses many medications to treat the same ailment or when an inappropriate drug is prescribed for the patient's condition. It can also happen when a person combines herbal remedies or dietary supplements with prescription drugs or when they take different pharmaceuticals simultaneously to treat various ailments with similar mechanisms of action. Older patients are one group that is particularly vulnerable to polypharmacy. To treat pain, constipation, sleeplessness and indigestion, they may take over-the-counter (OTC) medications. While polypharmacy may be required in some circumstances, such as when a patient needs to take several drugs to manage a chronic ailment, it raises the possibility of negative side effects and pharmaceutical interactions. Children, those with mental problems and older patients are all impacted by this problem. The increased risk of polypharmacy can be attributed to a number of factors, such as frequent use of OTC medications, medication ignorance and misguided drug perception.

To minimize the risks associated with polypharmacy, health care providers must work together to ensure that the patient's medication regimen is as simple as possible. This can be done by regularly reviewing the patient's medication list, making adjustments as necessary and reducing the number of medications and potential drug interactions. Consider alternative treatment options too, such as physical therapy or lifestyle changes, before prescribing multiple medications.

Safe Drug Management and Disposal

Safe drug management and disposal are critical components of reducing the risk of medication-related issues, such as polypharmacy, adverse drug reactions and medication errors. Drug stewardship is one aspect of safe drug management, which involves ensuring that medications are used appropriately and that patients are receiving the right medications for their specific needs. This can be achieved through several methods, such as:

Regular medication reviews – Health care providers should regularly review patients' medication lists to identify any potential issues, such as duplicate medications, drug interactions or unnecessary medications.

Monitoring for adverse reactions – Health care providers should closely monitor patients for any adverse reactions to their medications and adjust the treatment plan as necessary.

Medication reconciliation – This process involves comparing patients' medication lists to the medications that are prescribed and administered to them, which helps ensure that patients are receiving the correct medications and there are no discrepancies between the medications that are prescribed and those a patient is taking at home.

Home medication management is another important aspect of safe drug management, which consists of educating patients on how to properly store, use and dispose of their medications.

Teach patients how to:

1. Recognize and report adverse reactions.
2. Communicate with their health care providers about their medications.
3. Follow the correct dosage and administration instructions.
4. Store the medication in appropriate conditions.

Drug disposal, on the other hand, refers to the safe disposal of medications that are no longer needed or have expired. This includes:

- Taking unused or expired medications to a medication take-back program or a designated disposal site
- Avoiding flushing medications down the toilet or throwing them in the trash, as this can contaminate the water supply and harm wildlife
- Following the disposal instructions on the medication label or asking a health care provider or pharmacist for guidance

Pain Management

Chronic and/or Acute Pain Management

Pain management is a critical aspect of health care, and assessing pain is the first step in developing an effective treatment plan. Various tools and methods can be used to assess pain, including subjective pain assessment tools, visual aids, questionnaires and observing for objective signs.

One commonly used tool for assessing pain is the 0-to-10 rating scale. Assessing pain allows patients to rate the severity of their discomfort on a numerical scale, where 0 represents the absence of pain and 10 represents the most intense pain imaginable. This simple and easy-to-use method can be used to monitor the effectiveness of pain management interventions over time.

Another tool is the face-rating scale. This method uses illustrations of different facial expressions to help patients communicate the intensity and nature of their pain. By selecting the face that most closely represents their pain sensation, patients can help health care providers gauge the effectiveness of interventions and make necessary adjustments.

Other methods of pain assessment include questionnaires, body diagrams and pain flow charts, which can provide more detailed information about the location, intensity and quality of a patient's pain, as well as any factors that relieve or worsen it.

Objective signs of pain, such as facial grimacing, elevated blood pressure, increased pulse and respiratory rates, muscle tension, restlessness, decreased interest in surroundings, perspiration, pallor, crying, moaning or verbalizing pain and guarding the painful body part, can also be used to assess pain.

Pain can be classified into two categories: acute and chronic. Acute pain is mild to severe pain that has a rapid onset and lasts less than six months. Chronic pain, on the other hand, lasts beyond the expected healing time and may be challenging to relate to the original injury or tissue damage.

Pharmacological and Nonpharmacological

Acute pain management typically involves the use of medications, such as nonsteroidal anti-inflammatory drugs (NSAIDs), acetaminophen and opioid analgesics. These medications can be administered orally, parenterally (such as subcutaneously, intramuscularly and intravenously), intraspinally (epidurally) and topically. Nurses may also assist with the administration of regional anesthesia techniques, such as epidurals, spinal blocks and nerve blocks, as well as with patient-controlled analgesia (PCA) systems and scheduled dosing regimens.

For chronic pain management, the implementation of nonpharmacologic interventions, such as physical therapy, cognitive-behavioral therapy and occupational therapy, is crucial. Those interventions can be accompanied by medications, such as antidepressants, anticonvulsants and muscle relaxants, and the administration of transcutaneous electrical nerve stimulation (TENS) and spinal cord stimulation.

In addition to administering medications and implementing interventions, nurses play an important role in educating patients and their families about pain management strategies and monitoring the effectiveness of treatments. They should also be aware of the potential side effects of medications and the importance of individualized pain management plans that consider patients' specific needs and preferences.

Multimodal Approach

Multimodal pain management refers to the use of multiple modalities or interventions to manage pain rather than relying on a single approach. This approach can include a combination of pharmacologic and nonpharmacologic interventions to target different aspects of the pain experience.

For acute pain management, a multimodal approach may include the use of NSAIDs, acetaminophen and opioid analgesics in combination with regional anesthesia techniques, such as epidurals, spinal blocks and nerve blocks, as well as PCA systems and scheduled dosing regimens. Nonpharmacological interventions, such as ice, heat and relaxation techniques, can also be used.

For chronic pain management, a multimodal approach may include the use of medications, such as antidepressants, anticonvulsants and muscle relaxants, in combination with physical therapy, cognitive-behavioral therapy and occupational therapy. Nerve blocks, TENS and spinal cord stimulation may also be used.

The capacity to target different pain pathways, lower the risk of side effects and enhance pain control are all advantages of a multimodal strategy. Additionally, it enables the creation of personalized treatment programs that take the patient's particular requirements and preferences into account.

Patient Pain Management Expectation

Depending on the person's unique condition, different patients may have different expectations for pain treatment. Nonetheless, a few typical goals that patients might have include:

1. **Effective pain management** – Patients expect that their pain will be well managed and that their level of discomfort will be significantly reduced.

2. **Timely pain relief** – Patients expect that their pain will be treated quickly and that they will not have to wait a long time to receive pain medication.

3. **Safety** – Patients expect that their pain treatment will be secure and low-risk in terms of negative effects.

4. **Communication** – Patients expect that their health care professionals will pay attention to their worries and provide them with a thorough explanation of their pain management strategy.

5. **Customized care** – Patients expect that their pain management strategy will be developed in accordance with their unique requirements and preferences.

6. **Ongoing assessment** – Patients expect that their pain will be monitored continuously and that their pain management strategy will be modified as necessary to maintain pain relief.

7. **Collaboration** – This is something that patients demand from their medical professionals in order to manage their pain and be a part of any decisions that are made regarding their care.

8. **Empathy** – Patients expect that their medical professionals will approach pain treatment with empathy and compassion.

Patient Advocacy

Promoting patients' rights and well-being while ensuring that their demands are satisfied in a secure and efficient manner is known as patient advocacy in the field of pain treatment. It entails attending to the patients' needs and comprehending their pain experience, clearly outlining their pain management plans, including patients in decision-making regarding their care, consistently assessing and modifying patients' pain management plans, effectively collaborating with the interdisciplinary team and being aware of and adhering to guidelines and protocols for pain management.

Nonpharmacological Interventions

Nonpharmacological pain management is a comprehensive method of pain control that makes use of nondrug techniques to reduce pain and enhance the patient's general well-being. These can involve a range of methods, such as complementary and alternative therapies, physical therapies and psychiatric therapies. For nurses, this may mean:

1. Monitoring patients' pain levels and making adjustments as necessary, such as repositioning, which helps lessen the discomfort by dispersing pressure, boosting circulation and encouraging relaxation

2. Informing patients and their families on the causes of pain, the advantages and drawbacks of various pain management techniques and self-management techniques

3. Making use of nonpharmacologic treatments, such as acupuncture, biofeedback, cutaneous stimulation, therapeutic touch, ice and heat therapy and cognitive and behavioral pain management

4. Encouraging patients to take an active role in their treatment, such as including them in the creation of a pain management strategy

5. Working with other members of the health care team to provide comprehensive pain treatment, including, when necessary, seeking the advice of pain experts, physical therapists and other specialists.

6. Recording and reporting the patients' level of discomfort, responsiveness to interventions and any negative effects.

Complementary and Alternative Therapies

Cutaneous stimulation, therapeutic touch, acupuncture, cognitive and behavioral pain management and biofeedback are some of the complementary alternative medicine (CAM) techniques that can be used to manage pain.

Cutaneous stimulation is a nonpharmacologic method of pain management that utilizes touch and pressure on the skin to alleviate pain and improve circulation. Heat therapy (thermotherapy) and cold therapy (cryotherapy) are used to stimulate the skin and underlying tissues, providing temporary relief from pain and discomfort. Heat therapy can increase blood flow and relax muscles, while cold therapy can reduce inflammation and numb the affected area.

Therapeutic touch is a form of energy healing that entails the practitioner using their hands to channel healing energy to the patient. The practitioner is thought to sense and manipulate the patient's energy field to promote healing and reduce pain.

Acupuncture, a traditional Chinese medicine practice, involves inserting needles into special points on the body. These points correspond to different pathways or channels in the body called meridians, which are believed to be connected to the flow of energy throughout the body. Stimulating these acupoints aims to balance the flow of energy and alleviate pain.

Cognitive and behavioral pain management focuses on using relaxation, visualization and mindfulness to manage pain rather than solely relying on medication.

Biofeedback enables an individual to control certain physiological processes, such as heart rate and muscle tension, to manage pain and other symptoms. This technique typically involves electronic sensors and monitoring equipment to provide the person with feedback on their physiological state. By learning to control these processes, the person can learn to reduce pain and other symptoms by changing the way they respond to stress and other triggers.

The repositioning effect is another nonpharmacologic intervention that can be used to manage pain by changing the position of the body. This can include repositioning a limb, changing the position of a joint or repositioning the entire body. Repositioning can help reduce pain by redistributing pressure, increasing circulation and promoting relaxation.

Aromatherapy uses essential oils from plants to promote physical and psychological well-being. Aromatherapy is believed to work by stimulating the olfactory system and activating certain areas of the brain associated with emotions, memories and physiological processes. Different essential oils have different therapeutic properties and are used for different purposes, such as lavender oil for relaxation and peppermint oil for headaches.

Surgical/Procedural Nursing Management

Pre- and Post-Procedural Unit Standards

Pre- and post-procedural unit standards are important guidelines that help ensure the safety and well-being of patients before, during and after a surgical procedure. For medical-surgical nurses, these standards may include:

Consent – Obtaining informed consent from the patient before the procedure. This includes explaining the procedure, its risks and benefits and any alternative options. The patient's signature on a consent form serves as documentation of the person's understanding and agreement to the procedure.

Timeout – A pause in the surgical procedure to ensure that the correct patient, procedure and site are being worked on. The surgical team will verbally confirm the patient's identity, the procedure to be performed and the surgical site before proceeding with the surgery.

Monitoring – Frequently monitoring the patient's vital signs and level of consciousness before, during and after the procedure. This includes monitoring the patient's heart rate, blood pressure, oxygen saturation and temperature, as well as any other vital signs that are relevant to the specific procedure.

Preparation and positioning – Preparing patients for surgery by placing them in the correct position for the procedure, ensuring that all necessary equipment and supplies are readily available and ensuring that patients are properly draped to maintain privacy and prevent infection.

Sterilization – Maintaining a sterile environment during the procedure, including following proper hand hygiene and sterilization protocols.

Medication administration – Administering appropriate medications as ordered by the surgeon to the patient, including preoperative medications and pain management medications.

Table 6. Medications

Class	Drug	Purpose
Antibiotics	Cefazolin (Ancef)	Prevent postoperative infection
Anticholinergics	Atropine (Isopto Atropine)	Reduce oral and respiratory secretions
Glycopyrrolate (Robinul)	Reduce secretions	
Scopolamine (Transderm-Scop)	Prevent nausea and vomiting	
Sedatives	Midazolam (Versed)	Induce sedation, antianxiety and amnesic effects
Diazepam (Valium)	Induce sedation and antianxiety	
Lorazepam (Ativan)	Induce sedation, antianxiety and amnesic effects	
Antidiabetics	Insulin (Humulin R)	Stabilize blood glucose
Antiemetics	Metoclopramide (Reglan)	Promote gastric emptying and prevent nausea and vomiting
Ondansetron (Zofran)	Prevent nausea and vomiting	
B-Blockers	Labetalol (Normodyne)	Manage hypertension
Histamine H2-Receptor Antagonists	Famotidine (Pepcid)	Reduce acid secretion and gastric volume

Opioids	Morphine (Duramorph)	Relieve pain during preoperative procedures
	Fentanyl (Sublimaze)	Relieve pain during preoperative procedures	

Recovery and postoperative care: The immediate aftermath of surgery is a critical time for patients, and the post-anesthesia care unit (PACU) is designed to provide close monitoring and care during this period. Located adjacent to the operating room (OR), the PACU allows for easy access to anesthesia and OR personnel, minimizing the need for transportation and ensuring that patients promptly receive the care they need. The level of care provided in the PACU is tailored to the patient's individual needs and is divided into three phases. Upon admission to the PACU, the patient's care is a collaborative effort between the anesthesia care provider (ACP), the OR nurse and the PACU nurse.

The patient's condition will determine how the person progresses through the different phases of care, with stable and recovering patients potentially able to move quickly through Phase I to discharge or transfer to Phase II care or an inpatient unit.

Patient Post-Surgery Assessment

The first step in post-surgery patient care is to assess the patient's airway, breathing and circulation (ABC) status. During the initial assessment, any signs of inadequate oxygenation and ventilation should be identified and treated promptly. One useful tool for monitoring oxygenation is pulse oximetry, which provides a noninvasive means of measuring oxygen levels in the blood.

Additionally, transcutaneous carbon dioxide and end-tidal CO_2 monitoring (capnography) can be used to detect respiratory depression. It is also important to note and evaluate any deviations in the patient's electrocardiographic results from preoperative findings and to measure and compare the patient's blood pressure with the baseline readings. Invasive monitoring may be initiated if needed.

Other important aspects of the initial assessment include evaluating the patient's body temperature, capillary refill and skin condition, as well as assessing the level of consciousness orientation and sensory and motor function.

For patients who have received a regional anesthetic, such as a spinal or epidural, it is important to check for any residual sensory or motor blockade and to explain all activities to the patient from the moment of admission to the PACU. Additionally, the patient's urinary system should be assessed for intake, output and fluid balance. This includes noting the presence of all IV lines, irrigation solutions and output devices, such as catheters and wound drains. Finally, it is important to implement any postoperative orders related to incision care, such as monitoring the surgical site and managing any dressings or drainage.

Communication – Communicating with the surgical team, the patient and the patient's family throughout the procedure, including providing updates on the patient's condition, addressing any concerns and providing instructions for postoperative care.

Pertinent Potential Complications and Management

Operating Room (OR) Emergencies

Although extensive planning and preparation go into surgeries, unexpected events can still happen despite the best efforts. These occurrences can be predicted, like a cardiac arrest in a seriously unwell patient, or wholly unexpected, like massive blood loss during a trauma surgery. Malignant hyperthermia and anaphylactic responses are two instances of such unplanned outcomes. Both situations call for swift and firm action from the entire surgical team in order to lessen the risk of patient injury. All members of the OR team must be aware of these kinds of emergencies and be ready to act promptly and efficiently should they arise.

A severe, sometimes fatal allergic reaction called anaphylaxis can happen during surgery. It is brought on by a number of things, including adverse effects from injections of anesthetics, antibiotics, blood products and other substances. Low blood pressure, a rapid heartbeat, bronchospasm and potential fluid buildup in the lungs are all signs of an allergic reaction. The surgical team must be aware of the possibility of an anaphylactic reaction and be ready to act immediately if it does occur.

Due to the widespread use of latex-containing products, like gloves and catheters, latex allergy is becoming an increasing concern in the surgical field. From minor skin irritation to severe anaphylactic reactions, latex can cause a variety of reactions. Symptoms can arise at any point during the operation. Hospitals and other health care institutions must have policies in place to guarantee a latex-free environment in order to safeguard patients who have latex allergies.

Table 7. Treatment of Anaphylactic Reaction During Surgery

Step	Action
1	Stop the administration of the suspected allergen.
2	Administer epinephrine (1:1,000) intramuscularly or subcutaneously.
3	Administer antihistamines, such as diphenhydramine (Benadryl).
4	Administer steroids, such as prednisolone or methylprednisolone.
5	Administer bronchodilators, such as albuterol, to relieve bronchospasm.
6	Administer oxygen to maintain adequate oxygenation.
7	Administer IV fluids to maintain blood pressure and treat shock.
8	Monitor vital signs, including blood pressure, heart rate and oxygen saturation.
9	If symptoms persist or worsen, consider the administration of epinephrine through continuous infusion or repeated doses.
10	Notify the patient's primary care physician and the patient's allergist, if available.

Note that the above table serves as a general guideline; specific treatment protocols may vary based on the patient's condition, the severity of the reaction and the availability of medication. Also, the treatment may need to be adapted according to the patient's vital signs and the presence of any associated complications. The most important step is to stop the administration of the suspected allergen as soon as possible.

Malignant hyperthermia is a rare but potentially fatal disorder that occurs when certain anesthetic agents are administered to susceptible individuals. It is characterized by a rapid increase in body temperature, muscle rigidity and other metabolic changes. It is essential for medical professionals to be aware of the possibility of malignant hyperthermia and to take appropriate precautions, such as obtaining a detailed family history and being alert for signs of the disorder during surgery. The treatment of malignant hyperthermia is the immediate administration of dantrolene.

Postoperative Complications

Table 8. Postoperative Complications and Treatment for Medical-Surgical Nurses

Complication	Description	Treatment
Hematoma	Blood collecting outside blood vessels	Drainage of the area using a needle and syringe or small incision. Administration of blood thinners, such as heparin or warfarin. In some cases, a pressure dressing may be applied to reduce swelling.
Infection	Microorganisms entering the surgical site	Wound drainage, antibiotics and reopening the surgical site if necessary. A wound vacuum or vacuum-assisted closure device may be used to remove infected material and promote healing.
Blood clot	Blood clot forming in the veins of the legs or lungs	Blood thinners, such as heparin or warfarin, compression stockings and physical therapy to improve circulation and prevent blood clots from forming.
Nerve injury	Injury to nerves near the surgical site	Physical therapy, nerve blocks and, in severe cases, reoperation to repair or reconstruct the damaged nerve.
Anesthesia complications	Reactions to anesthesia or difficulty breathing	Oxygen therapy, medication and, in severe

		cases, intubation to maintain an open airway.
Wound breakdown	The surgical incision opens or becomes infected.	Wound care, antibiotics and reopening the surgical site if necessary to remove infected or necrotic tissue.
Scarring	Abnormal or excessive scarring at the surgical site	Topical creams, such as silicone gel or onion extract, silicone sheeting, and, in severe cases, revision surgery to remove or revise the scar.

Medical-surgical nurses closely monitor the patient's condition, vital signs and wound healing and promptly report and document any signs of complications to the surgeon. Nursing care should be individualized based on the patient's needs and the surgeon's postoperative instructions.

Scope of Practice Related to Procedures

The scope of practice for medical-surgical nurses includes a wide range of responsibilities related to the care of patients before, during and after surgical procedures. Some specific responsibilities include:

1. Assessing patient needs and developing a care plan
2. Administering medication, including preoperative and postoperative medication
3. Monitoring vital signs, such as blood pressure, heart rate and oxygen levels
4. Providing patient education and emotional support
5. Assisting the surgeon during the procedure
6. Maintaining a sterile environment in the operating room
7. Documenting patient information and progress
8. Collaborating with other members of the health care team, such as physicians and other nurses, to ensure the best possible care
9. Administering sedation and monitoring the patient's level of sedation and vital signs during the procedure.

Moderate sedation, also referred to as conscious sedation, is achieved through the administration of sedative, hypnotic and opioid drugs via an IV route. This includes etomidate, diazepam, midazolam, fentanyl, alfentanil, propofol and morphine sulfate.

Sedation is frequently used in short medical procedures that require pain management, such as endoscopies, cardiac catheterization and fracture reduction. Patient's vitals, including the level of consciousness, oxygen levels, heart rate and airway, are closely monitored every 15 to 30 minutes during and after the procedure.

The American Society of Anesthesiologists (ASA) has a protocol for nurses administering sedation called the ASA Sedation Guidelines. The guidelines include the following steps:

Table 9. ASA Sedation Guidelines

Step	Details
1	**Pre-procedure assessment**
	- Medical history
	- Medications
	- Allergies
	- Current condition
2	**Selection of appropriate level of sedation**
	- Patient's condition
	- Procedure being performed
	- Patient's preferences
3	**Continuous monitoring**
	- Vital signs
	- Level of consciousness
	- Respiratory status
4	**Use of appropriate medication**
	- Select medication based on the patient's condition and level of sedation desired.
	- Medications should be titrated to the desired level of sedation.

5	**Recovery**	
		- Monitor patients until they have fully recovered from sedation and can resume normal activities.
6	**Documentation**	
		- Type of medication used
		- Dosage
		- Level of sedation achieved
		- Any adverse reactions

Supplies, Instruments and Equipment

Table 10. Medical-Surgical Nurse Equipment Overview

Category	Description
PPE	Gloves, gowns, masks, goggles or face shields and head covers to protect the nurse and the patient from infection
Surgical instruments	Scalpels, forceps, retractors, scissors, needle holders and hemostats used for performing procedures
Medical devices	Catheters, drains, feeding tubes and other equipment used for patient care
Medications and anesthesia	Medications, such as antibiotics, pain medications and blood thinners, as well as equipment and drugs used for anesthesia
Monitoring equipment	Blood pressure cuffs, pulse oximeters, thermometers and electrocardiograms (ECGs) to track vital signs
Sterilization equipment	Autoclaves and other equipment used to clean and disinfect instruments
Rehabilitation equipment	Exercise machines, walkers and crutches used to aid in patient recovery

47

Nutrition

Individualized Nutritional Needs

A well-rounded and balanced diet can provide the body with the essential nutrients it needs to function properly, while deficiencies or imbalances can lead to a host of health problems.

Unfortunately, as many as 50% of medical-surgical patients may suffer from moderate malnutrition, which can lead to significant health complications. The risk of malnutrition increases with the length of hospitalization, making early identification and intervention crucial.

One of the most critical steps in preventing malnutrition is conducting a thorough nutritional assessment. This assessment should include a patient's dietary history, which should cover typical consumption, eating patterns and preferences, use of supplements and any recent changes in appetite or conditions that may interfere with food ingestion or digestion.

To ensure the patient's diet aligns with the dietary guidelines outlined by the US Department of Agriculture's Food Guide Pyramid, health care providers should compare the information obtained from the dietary history with these guidelines. Additionally, the patient's height and weight should be measured, and the body mass index (BMI) should be calculated. A BMI value of less than 18.5 indicates malnutrition, while a value greater than 25 indicates overnutrition.

$$BMI = weight\ (kg)\ /\ height\ (m)^2$$

or

$$BMI = weight\ (lb)\ /\ height\ (in)^2 \times 703$$

Malnutrition

The clinical signs of malnutrition in adults are:

1. Weight loss
2. Muscle wasting
3. Fatigue
4. Decreased immune function
5. Anemia
6. Edema (swelling)
7. Dry and thinning hair
8. Brittle nails
9. Dry and scaly skin
10. Decreased wound healing
11. Irritability or apathy
12. Changes in mental status

Table 11. Malnutrition Markers and Indications

Markers	Indication
Visceral proteins (albumin, transferrin, prealbumin, retinol-binding protein)	Diminished levels indicate malnutrition.
Hemoglobin and hematocrit	Decreased levels indicate anemia, a common complication of malnutrition.
Vitamin and mineral levels (vitamin B12, folate, iron, zinc, selenium)	Low levels indicate specific nutrient deficiencies.
Inflammation markers (C-reactive protein)	Elevated levels indicate malnutrition.

Nitrogen balance is a measure of the adequacy of protein intake in the body. This can be determined by measuring protein intake in conjunction with 24-hour urinary urea nitrogen levels. When the loss of nitrogen exceeds the intake, it is considered a negative nitrogen balance, which is an indication of protein deficiency.

Negative nitrogen balance is often seen in malnutrition, chronic illness and injury. It is important to monitor nitrogen balance to ensure that individuals are receiving the appropriate amount of protein in their diet and to detect and address any deficiencies early on.

Table 12. Malnutrition Risks for Medical-Surgical Patients

Malnutrition Risks for Medical-Surgical Patients	Details
Malabsorption syndromes	Celiac disease, Crohn's disease and cystic fibrosis can make it difficult for the body to absorb nutrients properly, increasing the risk of malnutrition.
Gastric or bowel resections	Surgical procedures that involve the removal of part of the stomach or intestines can make it difficult for the body to absorb nutrients properly, increasing the risk of malnutrition.
Pancreatic insufficiency	Chronic pancreatitis, pancreatic cancer and cystic fibrosis can cause the pancreas to produce insufficient enzymes, making it difficult for the body to digest and absorb nutrients properly, increasing the risk of malnutrition.
Chronic medical conditions	Many chronic medical conditions, such as cancer, heart failure, kidney disease and diabetes, can increase the risk of malnutrition due to increased energy and nutrient requirements, decreased appetite and increased metabolic rate.
Increased blood loss, wound drainage and dialysis	These can lead to increased nutrient loss and decreased nutrient absorption, increasing the risk of malnutrition.
Increased nutrient needs due to stress response, cancer, surgery, infection, trauma and burns	This can lead to increased nutrient loss and decreased nutrient absorption, increasing the risk of malnutrition.
Medications causing side effects, such as nausea, vomiting and loss of appetite	Some medications, such as cisplatin, morphine, fentanyl, metoclopramide, dronabinol, haloperidol, risperidone, etc., can contribute to malnutrition by decreasing appetite and nutrient absorption.

Therapeutic Diets

Clear liquid diets – These diets are designed for patients who need a low-residue diet before or after a medical procedure. They consist of clear liquids, such as water, broth, clear juices, tea and soda. They are used for a short period, as they provide inadequate nutrition for long-term use.

Full liquid diets – These diets are a step up from clear liquid diets. They include milk, milkshakes, yogurt, cream soups and liquid nutritional supplements. They are used as an intermediate step between clear liquid and soft diets to provide patients with the necessary nutrients while allowing the gastrointestinal tract to rest and recover.

Soft diets – This type of diet is suitable for patients who have difficulty swallowing or chewing. It includes foods that are easy to chew and swallow, such as pureed fruits and vegetables, mashed potatoes and cooked cereal.

Low-residue diets – This diet is designed for patients who have had bowel surgery or suffer from inflammatory bowel disease. It reduces the amount of fiber in the diet to decrease the amount of stool and gas produced.

Low-sodium diets – This diet is designed for patients who have heart failure or kidney disease or are on dialysis. It aims to decrease the amount of sodium in the diet to decrease the risk of fluid retention and hypertension.

Nutrition Administration Modalities

Enteral Nutrition

Enteral nutrition refers to the delivery of nutrient solutions directly into the stomach or small intestine through a tube that is inserted through the nose, mouth or directly into the stomach or small intestine through surgery. This method of nutrition administration is used when a person is unable to eat or drink enough to maintain their nutritional status, typically due to a medical condition, such as a chronic illness, injury or surgery that affects the gastrointestinal tract.

Table 13. Types of Enteral Nutrition

Types of Enteral Nutrition	Description
Continuous enteral nutrition	A steady, continuous flow of nutrition through the tube. Typically used for patients who are unable to eat or have a decreased appetite but still have an intact GI tract.
Bolus enteral nutrition	A larger volume of nutrition in smaller, more frequent doses. Typically used for patients who have a higher calorie requirement or are unable to tolerate continuous enteral nutrition.

Table 14. Types of Enteral Access

Types of Enteral Access	Description
Small-bore nasoenteric tube	Suitable for short-term enteral access lasting less than four weeks.
Gastroscopy or jejunostomy tube	Required for long-term enteral access lasting more than six weeks.

Before starting enteral nutrition, the placement of the tube must be confirmed by X-ray or, if inserted endoscopically, by direct visualization. Always follow infection-control guidelines and the facility's protocols for handling and discarding enteral nutrition products.

Complications

Table 15. Complications and Prevention

Complication	Prevention
Tube obstruction	Gently flush the tube with 30 mL of warm water before and after feedings.
Aspiration pneumonia	Elevate the head of the bed 30 degrees during feedings.
Dislocated nasoenteric tube	Check tube placement by X-ray or pH of gastric secretions.
Insertion site infection or leakage	Secure the tube to minimize trauma to the insertion site.
GI complications	Monitor for diarrhea, delayed gastric emptying and constipation.
Hyperglycemia	Monitor blood glucose levels.
Fluid and electrolyte imbalance	Monitor electrolyte levels and fluid intake and output.

Parenteral Nutrition

Parenteral nutrition, also known as IV nutrition, is a medical therapy that provides essential nutrients through IV infusion for patients who are unable to consume or absorb enough nutrition through oral or enteral means and require nutritional support for an extended period.

This method of nutrition delivery is typically recommended for patients who have a functional gastrointestinal tract and is used for less than 10 days. When it comes to parenteral nutrition, there are two main options for delivery: peripheral venous nutrition (PVN) and central venous nutrition (CVN).

PVN, also known as peripheral parenteral nutrition, is delivered through a peripheral vein, such as in the arm or hand. This method is typically used for patients who require short-term nutritional support for a period of up to two weeks. It is a less invasive option compared to CVN and can be administered in a hospital or outpatient setting.

CVN, also known as central parenteral nutrition, is delivered through a central vein, such as in the neck or chest. This method is typically used for patients who require long-term nutritional support, as it allows for more consistent and controlled delivery of nutrients. It is a more invasive option and is typically administered in a hospital setting.

Parenteral nutrition, whether delivered through PVN or CVN, consists of a combination of essential nutrients, including glucose, amino acids, electrolytes, vitamins and trace elements. However, the specific formulations and concentrations of these nutrients may vary between PVN and CVN.

PVN typically contains formulations with up to 10% glucose and less than 25% amino acids. These lower concentrations are suitable for short-term nutritional support through a peripheral vein. On the other hand, CVN is used for longer-term nutritional support and contains higher concentrations of glucose and amino acids that are infused centrally.

Parenteral nutrition can also include the use of fat emulsions, which provide essential fatty acids and can be administered through either peripheral or central veins. Additionally, total nutrient admixtures that contain a combination of proteins, carbohydrates and lipids in a single IV bag are also available.

Table 16. Types of Central Access Devices

Device	Description	Duration of use	Invasiveness
Non-tunneled or percutaneous catheter	Inserted at the bedside, typically used for short-term nutritional support	Up to a few weeks	Less invasive
Peripherally inserted central catheter (PICC)	Inserted through a peripheral vein, intended for short-term use	Up to a few weeks	More invasive than a non-tunneled catheter
Tunneled catheter (Hickman, Broviac, Groshong)	Inserted surgically, intended for long-term use	Long term	More invasive than a PICC
Implanted vascular access device	Surgically implanted, contains no external parts; access is through a special needle	Long term	Most invasive but most secure and long term

While parenteral nutrition can be an effective way to provide nutritional support, it is not without risks. Some of the most common complications associated with parenteral nutrition include:

- **Hypoglycemia and hyperglycemia** – Parenteral nutrition solutions often contain high levels of glucose, which can lead to imbalances in blood sugar levels.
- **Fluid overload** – Parenteral nutrition solutions are administered via an IV, which can lead to fluid accumulation in the body.
- **Electrolyte imbalances** – Parenteral nutrition solutions can disrupt the balance of electrolytes in the body, which can cause a variety of symptoms.
- **Infection** – Because the solutions used in parenteral nutrition are administered via a catheter, there is a risk of infection at the insertion site. Additionally, the high glucose and fat concentrations of the solutions can create an ideal environment for bacteria and fungi to grow.
- **Catheter complications** – Parenteral nutrition catheters can become occluded or dislodged, which can lead to a variety of complications.
- **Phlebitis** – Inflammation of the vein at the site of catheter insertion can occur.
- **Air embolism** – Parenteral nutrition solutions can cause air bubbles to form, which can travel to the lungs and cause an air embolism. If this is suspected, the patient should be positioned on the left side with the head down to allow bubbles to rise to the right atrium, where they are less likely to obstruct blood flow to the pulmonary artery.

Some important nursing actions to consider include:

- Assess all medical-surgical patients for nutritional status upon admission and at least weekly thereafter. This includes evaluating the patient's weight, BMI, dietary intake and any symptoms of malnutrition or malabsorption. If any deficits are detected, it is important to intervene as quickly as possible to address the issue.
- Provide individualized nutritional strategies for special populations, such as vegetarians, bariatric surgery patients and elderly patients. These populations have unique nutritional needs and require special attention to ensure they are getting the nutrients they need.
- Teach patients about maintaining a healthy diet at home before discharge. This should take into account the patient's food preferences and socioeconomic conditions.
- Check patients' weight and BMI regularly to help identify patients with obesity.
- Educate the patient and the family about the appropriate diet, physical activity and lifestyle changes that can help in achieving and maintaining a healthy weight.

- Refer patients with obesity to a dietitian or a nutritionist for an individualized nutrition plan.
- Monitor patients with obesity for the development of comorbidities, such as diabetes, hypertension and cardiovascular disease, and refer them for appropriate management.

For patients who will be administering parenteral nutrition at home, they and their caregivers must receive comprehensive education and support to ensure that they understand the equipment needed, how to properly care for the catheter and how to monitor for any potential complications. This includes teaching them how to properly handle and store the solutions, how to use the infusion pump and how to recognize and respond to any signs of complications, such as infection or catheter blockage.

Resources for Alternate Nutrition Administration

There are several resources available to help patients who are receiving alternate forms of nutrition. These can include:

Speech consultation – For individuals who are receiving enteral or parenteral nutrition and have difficulty swallowing, a speech therapist can provide exercises and techniques to improve swallowing function and reduce the risk of aspiration.

Dietary consultation – A registered dietitian can provide guidance on the composition of enteral and parenteral nutrition solutions and make recommendations for adjustments based on an individual's nutritional needs and medical conditions. They can also provide education on how to manage the diet and medications related to alternate nutrition administration.

Nurses and other health care professionals trained in the administration of enteral and parenteral nutrition can provide **education and support** for individuals receiving these forms of nutrition.

Home health care agencies can provide **equipment and supplies** for enteral and parenteral nutrition, as well as trained staff, to assist with administering these forms of nutrition in the home.

Indications for Alternate Nutrition Administration

Alternate forms of nutrition administration, such as enteral and parenteral nutrition, may be indicated in certain medical conditions or scenarios where a patient is unable to obtain adequate nutrition through oral intake alone. These include, but are not limited to:

1. Gastrointestinal disorders that affect the ability to absorb nutrients, such as Crohn's disease or severe short bowel syndrome
2. Neurological disorders that affect the ability to swallow, such as ALS or brain injury
3. Cancer treatment that causes a loss of appetite or severe nausea
4. Recovery from surgery or severe injury
5. Advanced stages of certain illnesses, such as AIDS, cancer and COPD
6. Chronic illnesses such as cachexia, anemia and malnutrition

Chapter 3: Holistic Patient Care

Patient-Centered Care

Patient-centered care is an approach to health care that focuses on the patient's needs, preferences and values. It emphasizes a collaborative relationship between the patient and health care provider and actively involves the patient in the decision-making process. This approach empowers patients to take an active role in their own care, which can lead to improved adherence to treatment plans and reduced medical errors.

Individualized Patient Care

Individualized care is a holistic approach that prioritizes each patient's unique needs. It involves understanding the patient's values, preferences and cultural background, along with tailoring the care provided to best meet those needs.

To achieve this, empathetic, two-way communication is essential, where the health care provider actively listens to and engages with the patient while also respecting the patient's privacy and values. Clear and effective communication is key to understanding the patient's needs and providing care that aligns with their goals.

Effective communication is a crucial aspect of individualized care, as it allows for a deeper understanding of the patient's needs and preferences. Each party to a clinical encounter brings their own unique perspectives, shaped by their past experiences, cultural heritage, religious beliefs, level of education and self-concept. These personal factors affect the way messages are sent and received. Nonverbal cues, such as body movement, facial expression, touch and eye movement, can often convey more than words.

To establish a trusting relationship with the patient, the medical-surgical nurse must make a conscious effort to exhibit compassion and empathy. This can be achieved by maintaining eye contact, using an open posture and actively listening. It is important to remember the golden rule of treating patients the way you would want to be treated in their situation.

One common mistake that health care professionals make is failing to listen carefully to the patient. Good listening skills require concentration and appropriate responses to the patient's comments and questions. Patients are able to quickly tell when active listening is absent and may interpret this as a lack of concern or empathy. It is best to ask the patient to explain a statement if there is something the nurse does not understand. Nonetheless, a number of things, including emotions, linguistic limitations, listening abilities and comfort levels, might have an impact on messaging.

These elements may hinder communication and make it challenging for the health care professional to properly comprehend the patient's demands. The patient's level of comfort can be impacted by such variables as temperature, lighting, noise and privacy, all of which have a big impact on communication. In addition to making it challenging for the patient to concentrate on speaking, this might cause nonverbal signs of discomfort, such as sighing, restlessness, staring into space and avoiding eye contact.

Health care professionals must be aware of these aspects and foster an atmosphere that encourages good communication. The active involvement of family members in the patient's health care experience is referred to as family involvement in patient-centered care. This can involve helping make decisions, offering emotional support and helping out with caregiving at home.

Including family members in care planning and treatment decisions, training them to administer medication or manage symptoms at home, providing them with information and resources to support the patient's health and including them in discussions about the patient's prognosis and end-of-life care are some examples of family involvement in patient care.

The defined, quantifiable and doable objectives that are set for patients to enhance their health and well-being are referred to as health goals in patient-centered care. These objectives are frequently created in conjunction with the patient. Managing symptoms, such as minimizing pain or maintaining blood sugar levels in diabetes; improving mental health, such as lowering anxiety or depression; and improving overall health and well-being, such as giving up smoking or adopting a healthier diet, are a few examples of health goals that may be established for a patient.

Health goals should be achievable. For example, "I want to reduce my blood sugar level" is a specific goal that can be measured by checking the blood sugar level and is achievable with proper treatment and lifestyle changes.

Guidelines for Patient-Centered Care

Table 17. The American Nurses Association (ANA) Guidelines for Patient-Centered Care

ANA guidelines for patient-centered care	Description
Respect for patient autonomy	Respect the patient's right to make decisions about their own care.
Partnership with patients and families	Work in partnership with patients and their families to develop care plans.
Compassionate care	Provide care that is kind, caring and sensitive to the patient's emotional and physical needs.
Coordination of care	Work with other members of the health care team to ensure that the patient receives coordinated and comprehensive care.
Cultural sensitivity	Be aware of and sensitive to the patient's cultural background and provide care that is respectful of the patient's cultural beliefs and practices.
Continuity of care	Provide care that is consistent over time and across different settings.
Patient and family education	Educate patients and families about health conditions and treatment options.

Resources for Patient-Centered Care

Resources can help patients stay informed about their health and aware of the assistance available to them once they are living independently. This can help patients take an active role in their own care and feel more in control of their health.

Personalized resources can be provided to patients by evaluating what resources best meet their individual needs. This can involve assessing the patient's medical history, current health status and individual preferences.

For example, a patient who has anxiety might benefit from information about therapy resources, such as counseling or support groups. A patient with a chronic condition, such as diabetes, might benefit from information about self-management resources, such as nutrition and exercise programs. A patient who is struggling with medication adherence might benefit from reminders and resources that help them keep track of their medication schedule.

Providing resources to patients can be done in various ways, such as through brochures, pamphlets, videos or online resources. Patients can also be directed to outside organizations or agencies that provide additional resources and support.

Patient Advocacy

This is discussed in detail earlier in the book.

Patient Satisfaction Management

Patient satisfaction is a measure of a patient's level of contentment with the health care services they receive. It is used as a benchmark to evaluate the quality of care a health care facility or provider offers. Factors that can affect patient satisfaction include the health care staff's availability and responsiveness, the facility's cleanliness and comfort, the treatment's effectiveness and the overall patient experience.

Surveys are commonly used to gather feedback from patients and may include questions about communication with providers, wait times and overall satisfaction with the care received. Measuring patient satisfaction helps health care organizations identify areas for improvement and assess the performance of individual providers.

The Joint Commission's guidelines on patient satisfaction measurement and improvement are based on the principle that patient satisfaction is a key indicator of the quality and safety of care health care organizations provide. By following these guidelines, health care organizations can ensure they are providing the highest quality care to their patients and continually striving to improve.

One of the key aspects of The Joint Commission's guidelines is the use of a standardized patient satisfaction survey. This survey should be validated and include questions about communication with providers, wait times and overall satisfaction with the care received. By regularly administering this survey, health care organizations can gather feedback from patients and use this information to identify areas in need of improvement. This may include making changes to the care provided, improving the patient experience or increasing staff.

Sharing results with staff and patients is also an important aspect of The Joint Commission's guidelines. By sharing the results of the patient satisfaction survey with staff, health care organizations can help staff understand how they are performing and motivate them to improve. By sharing the results with patients, health care organizations can help patients feel informed about the care they are receiving.

Regular collection and analysis of data are also important. By collecting and analyzing patient satisfaction data on a regular basis, health care organizations can track progress over time and identify trends or patterns in patient satisfaction.

The Joint Commission also recommends using patient satisfaction data in performance evaluations for individual providers and staff. This helps ensure that staff are held accountable for the care they provide and are motivated to improve patient satisfaction.

Finally, The Joint Commission recommends that health care organizations provide a mechanism for patients to file complaints and grievances and have a process in place to address them. This helps ensure that patients are heard and that issues are addressed in a timely and effective manner.

Satisfying patients can lead to better healing, fewer complaints, increased likelihood of returning and reduced likelihood of legal action.

Second Opinion

A second opinion can have a positive impact on patient satisfaction by providing increased confidence in diagnosis and treatment, improving communication and understanding, reducing anxiety and uncertainty and addressing the patient's concerns.

When providing a second opinion for patients, nurses may need to know the following information:

- The patient's medical history, including any previous diagnoses, treatments and medications
- The patient's current symptoms and concerns
- The patient's current test results and imaging studies
- Any previous treatment options that have been tried and the results of those treatments
- The patient's preferences and goals for treatment
- The patient's insurance and any financial considerations
- The patient's support system and availability of caregivers
- Any cultural or linguistic considerations that may impact the patient's care
- The patient's level of understanding and ability to participate in decision-making
- The availability and referral process for the specialist providing the second opinion

This information can help the specialist providing the second opinion make an informed decision about the patient's diagnosis and treatment options.

Service Recovery

Service recovery is the process of addressing and resolving problems that have occurred during a patient's experience with a health care organization. Service recovery is an important aspect of patient satisfaction management, as it can help mitigate the negative effects of a poor experience and prevent future problems from arising.

Service recovery can include a variety of steps, such as:

- **Identifying the problem** – The first step in service recovery is identifying the problem. This can be done through patient feedback or by monitoring and tracking incidents.
- **Apologizing** – A sincere apology can go a long way in mitigating the negative effects of a poor experience. It shows the patient that the health care organization recognizes and takes responsibility for the problem.
- **Providing compensation** – Depending on the nature of the problem, providing compensation to the patient can be an effective way to show that the health care organization values the patient's experience.
- **Fixing the problem** – The most important step in service recovery is taking action to fix the problem. This can involve changing policies and procedures or retraining staff to prevent similar problems from occurring in the future.
- **Following up** – It is always a good idea to follow up with the patient to ensure that the problem has been resolved to their satisfaction and they are satisfied with the service recovery process.
- **Service recovery** – This is an essential component of patient satisfaction management, as it can help reduce the negative effects of a poor experience and prevent future problems from arising. It can also improve the relationship between the patient and the health care organization.

Complaints and Grievances

Patient feedback, in the form of complaints and grievances, is a key aspect of health care delivery. Understanding the distinction between the two is vital for effective management and resolution. Complaints, as outlined by the Centers for Medicare & Medicaid Services (CMS), usually pertain to minor issues, such as room cleanliness or food preferences. These types of complaints can be quickly and efficiently resolved by staff present at the time of the incident and do not necessitate a written response from the facility. However, it is crucial to document the complaint and the actions taken to resolve it for the purpose of quality improvement.

Contrarily, grievances are formal or informal written or verbal complaints regarding patient care, abuse or neglect; issues related to the hospital's compliance with regulations; or Medicare billing. These types of feedback may be submitted during or after the patient's care and may be filed by the patient or the representative.

Diversity and Inclusion

Cultural and Linguistic Needs

Cultural understanding shapes the way patients perceive their health and illness. Nurses and other health care professionals must be aware of their patients' cultural backgrounds to provide effective and appropriate care.

Culture is a complex and multifaceted concept that includes various elements, such as beliefs, values, customs, norms, habits, language, thoughts and ways of life. It is acquired and passed down through generations, primarily within families and social organizations and is shared by most members of the group.

Cultural diversity encompasses the many differences among people, which can be visible or invisible. For example, a person's race describes visible physical characteristics, such as skin color, head shape and hair texture, while ethnicity describes a group's common social customs, values and beliefs. A person's race does not always determine ethnicity, and individuals from the same race may have different customs and beliefs. For instance, a white person of Russian descent may have different customs and beliefs about health care or family roles than a white person of Italian descent. It is important to note that assuming that all Black people come from an African background and referring to them as "African American" is not culturally competent.

Cultural competence is health care professionals' ability to provide care that is sensitive to the cultural and linguistic needs of patients from diverse backgrounds. This includes understanding and respecting the cultural backgrounds, beliefs and practices of patients and their families, as well as providing culturally appropriate care. It is important to recognize that cultural sensitivity, which refers to the ability to recognize and respect cultural differences, is not enough. Health care professionals must also possess the knowledge and skills they need to provide culturally appropriate care.

The NCSBN has developed guidelines for cultural and linguistic competency for nurses. These guidelines include the following key principles:

1. **Respect for diversity** – Nurses should recognize and respect the diversity of patients and their families and be aware of the impact of culture on health and illness.

2. **Cultural humility** – Nurses should be open to learning about their patients' language and cultural backgrounds and make an effort to comprehend and value their viewpoints.
3. **Language access** – Nurses should be able to support patients and their families with their language needs by using either interpreters or translated materials.
4. **Effective communication** – Communicating with patients and families requires nurses to be aware of their cultural and language backgrounds.
5. **Patient-centered care** – Nurses should give patients individualized treatment that is based on their requirements while also taking into account their linguistic and cultural backgrounds.
6. **Continuous learning** – By continuing their education and professional development, nurses should continuously work to increase their cultural and linguistic proficiency.

These principles can be applied as a framework to create policies and procedures in health care organizations and are designed to help nurses provide patients with care that is both culturally and linguistically appropriate.

The following are examples of cultural and linguistic needs of patients:

Sign languages – People who have hearing loss or are hard of hearing utilize sign languages. To transmit meaning, these languages combine hand gestures, facial expressions and body language. To connect with health care professionals, patients who use sign languages may need sign language interpreters or video remote interpreting services.

Oral languages – These may be expressed verbally or in writing. To connect with health care practitioners and comprehend their health issues and treatment options, patients who speak languages other than the one used in the health care context may need interpreter services or materials that have been translated into their native tongue.

Written languages – Text is used to transmit information via written languages in books, signage or other written materials. To comprehend their health conditions and treatment options, patients who are literate in a particular language may need written resources in that language, such as patient education materials, consent forms and appointment reminders.

Cultural and Linguistic Resources

Cultural and linguistic resources for patients refer to materials and services that are designed to support patients from diverse cultural and linguistic backgrounds in their health care experience. Some examples include:

Translated materials – Multilingual patient education materials, consent forms and appointment reminders are available. In a language they can comprehend, this can help patients understand their medical conditions, available treatments and the health care system.

Interpreter services – These services enable patients who speak other languages to communicate with health care professionals efficiently over the phone or in person. With the use of these services, patients may be given precise and useful care.

Multilingual staff – The presence of multilingual staff members might be viewed as a cultural and linguistic resource. They can help remove language barriers and offer patients a more welcoming and pleasant health care experience.

Culturally sensitive care – Patients can feel appreciated and included in their health care experience by receiving care that is attentive to their cultural and language needs.

Cultural competency training – Training health care professionals in cultural competency can help them recognize potential prejudices, appreciate and respect cultural differences and actively seek out opportunities to learn about other cultures.

Implicit Bias

Implicit bias refers to the unconscious attitudes or stereotypes that can influence our perceptions, attitudes and behaviors toward certain groups of people. These prejudices may be based on race, ethnicity, gender, sexual orientation and socioeconomic class, among other things. The attitudes and opinions that people are aware of and can control frequently differ from implicit biases.

Implicit bias in health care can result in differences in the level of patient care provided. For instance, a health care professional could unwittingly harbor prejudices about particular racial or ethnic groups, which might result in a lack of trust and communication between the provider and the patient and lower-than-expected care. In addition, health care professionals' decisions on a diagnosis and course of treatment may be impacted by implicit bias.

Implicit bias might cause medical professionals to ignore some patients' symptoms or diagnoses, or it might cause them to treat patients differently, depending on their race, ethnicity or other characteristics. Health care providers can receive training on cultural competence and awareness of their own biases, can work to develop a patient-centered approach and actively seek out diverse perspectives. Meanwhile, health care organizations can put policies and procedures in place to promote diversity, equity and inclusion to lessen the effects of implicit bias in health care.

Education of Patients and Families

Health Maintenance and Disease Prevention

Health maintenance refers to the actions and responsibilities that promote and support the health and well-being of patients. For nurses, this includes:

- Evaluating the patient's health status, identifying risk factors and creating treatment plans to address them
- Teaching patients and their families how to incorporate healthy habits, like regular exercise, eating a balanced diet and getting enough sleep, into their everyday lives
- Giving immunizations to patients and urging them to get vaccinated to stop the spread of infectious diseases
- Screening for prevalent illnesses, including cancer and heart disease and, if necessary, directing patients to the proper follow-up care
- Putting in place infection-control procedures, such as handwashing and the use of PPE, to stop the spread of infectious diseases in hospital settings
- Evaluating and taking care of patients' behavioral health requirements, such as those related to mental health and substance misuse, as part of all-encompassing treatment
- Coordinating care and communicating effectively with other health care providers to ensure continuity of care
- Encouraging patient self-management and self-care and providing education and resources to patients and families to take an active role in their health
- Keeping up with evidence-based practice and guidelines, updating knowledge and skills and participating in continuing education programs to stay current in the field

The ANA has several guidelines and recommendations related to health maintenance and disease prevention.

Table 18. ANA Guidelines

ANA Guidelines	Description
Promoting healthy lifestyles	The ANA encourages nurses to educate patients and the public about the importance of healthy behaviors, such as regular exercise, good nutrition and adequate sleep.
Screening and early detection	The ANA encourages nurses to advocate for and educate patients about the importance of regular screenings and early detection of common diseases, such as cancer and heart disease.
Immunization	The ANA supports the use of vaccines as a safe and effective way to prevent the spread of infectious diseases and encourages nurses to educate patients about the importance of vaccination.
Infection control	The ANA recommends that nurses follow infection-control guidelines to prevent the spread of infectious diseases in health care settings, including the use of PPE and standard precautions.
Behavioral health	The ANA encourages nurses to assess and address patients' behavioral health needs, including mental health and substance abuse, as part of comprehensive care.
Advocacy	The ANA encourages nurses to advocate for policies that support health maintenance and disease prevention, such as access to affordable health care, healthy food options and safe housing.

Health Literacy

Health literacy, as defined by the WHO, is an individual's ability to comprehend, interpret and act on health information in order to make informed decisions and take appropriate actions to maintain and improve their health.

It not only encompasses the cognitive skills of reading and understanding health information, but also includes the ability to apply that information in a meaningful way through personal actions and choices.

Health literacy is important for nurses to consider when interacting with patients. They should assess the patient's health literacy level; communicate in a clear, simple language; and provide written materials that are easy to read and understand. They should also encourage patients to ask questions and to participate in their care.

Additionally, nurses should be aware of cultural and linguistic diversity, as it can affect health literacy levels. They should take into account the patient's background, communication style and any language or cultural barriers that may exist.

Teaching Methods

Patient education involves a dynamic process of assessment, planning, implementation and evaluation. The approach used in patient teaching is similar to that of the nursing process, utilizing a problem-solving method to address the patient's needs and learning abilities.

The process is continuous, requiring health care professionals to continuously assess and evaluate the patient's understanding and progress in order to adapt their teaching strategies as needed. This approach allows for a personalized and effective educational experience, ensuring that the patient is empowered to take an active role in their own health and well-being.

Process of Education

The educational process is a vital component of health care that focuses on creating and implementing a teaching plan tailored to the patient's and family's needs. This process begins with assessing the patient's current level of knowledge, reading ability and learning style, as well as the perceived need for education.

This information is then used to develop a teaching plan that outlines clear learning objectives, relevant content and effective teaching methods. During the implementation of the teaching plan, the nurse must document activities and monitor progress to ensure that any necessary adjustments are made in a timely manner. The effectiveness of the teaching can be evaluated by testing skills through return demonstrations, creating hypothetical scenarios to gauge the patient's response and allowing the patient to explain their understanding of the topic. If further education is required, the nurse can refer the patient to additional resources within the community.

Documentation

Documentation is an essential aspect of the educational process in health care. The nurse is responsible for keeping detailed records of all teaching activities, including any instances when the patient is not ready to learn due to difficulty coping with an illness, uncontrolled pain or other factors. This documentation serves as a record of the patient's progress and can be used to make adjustments to the teaching plan as needed.

The nurse should also document the data used to assess the patient and the actions taken as a result of the assessment. This documentation not only serves as a record of the patient's progress but also provides valuable information for other health care professionals involved in the patient's care.

Practical Aspect

The practical aspects of teaching involve nurses' ability to effectively and efficiently utilize their time to meet patients' and families' educational needs. Teaching by nurses can be informal and may occur while the nurse performs other activities.

Incorporating patient and family input into the educational process is important for achieving long-term success. By engaging patients in discussions about their educational needs, nurses can build a sense of ownership and responsibility for their own learning. This approach can lead to more effective and efficient use of nursing time. To meet patients' and families' diverse learning needs, nurses can use creative methods, such as waiting room teaching sessions, printed materials and other multimedia resources. These methods allow nurses to provide targeted and relevant education in a variety of settings, increasing the chances that the patient will retain and apply the information learned.

Before patients are discharged, the nurse must ensure that they are aware of critical information pertaining to their condition and document this in the medical record. This is an important aspect of the educational process, as it ensures patients have the necessary information and skills to manage their condition and maintain their health after discharge.

Health Promotion

Health Promotion Goals

Health promotion is vital for nursing care, and nurses have a pivotal role in empowering individuals, families and communities to make well-informed decisions regarding their health and well-being. The WHO defines health promotion as the process of giving individuals the tools and resources they need to improve their health and increase control over it. As experienced and educated health care professionals, nurses are uniquely equipped to facilitate this process by delivering accurate and pertinent health information through health education and instruction.

Nurses are often the first point of contact for patients, and their expertise allows them to assess patients' health risks and develop care plans to address them. They also provide information and resources to help patients access community health services and advocate for policies and programs that promote health and prevent disease. In addition, nurses collaborate with other health care professionals and community organizations to improve the overall health of populations. Nurses can employ various strategies to achieve this goal, including primary, secondary and tertiary prevention.

Primary prevention is focused on preventing the onset of specific diseases by reducing risk factors through education and protection. For example, nurses may educate patients on the dangers of smoking and advocate for policies that restrict smoking in public places to reduce the risk of respiratory disease.

Secondary prevention includes procedures that detect and treat preclinical pathological changes, thereby controlling disease progression. Nurses may perform screening procedures, such as mammography, to detect early-stage breast cancer or routine blood sugar testing for people over 45 to facilitate early interventions.

Tertiary prevention aims to reduce the disability or complications arising from a condition and improve a patient's function, longevity and quality of life. Nurses may provide cardiac rehabilitation following a myocardial infarction, which may involve encouraging patients to alter their behaviors, such as losing weight, to reduce the likelihood of future occurrences.

The following table illustrates the various responsibilities that nurses have in promoting health and well-being.

Table 19. Nurses' Responsibilities in Health Promotion

Responsibilities	Description
Provide health information and advice about healthy lifestyles	Nurses provide valuable information and advice about healthy lifestyles to patients as the first point of contact.
Promote health promotion encounters	Nurses strive to make every encounter with a patient a health promotion encounter by assessing patients' health risks and developing care plans to address them.
Empower patients	Nurses aim to empower patients to feel more confident and competent in managing their health by developing personal skills that enable patients to take control of their health.
Facilitate access and use of the health care system	Nurses make health care more accessible and user-friendly by helping patients navigate the health care system and understand their health coverage options.
Promote social change and address inequalities	Nurses play a critical role in promoting social change and addressing inequalities by advocating for policies and programs that promote health and prevent disease and collaborating with other health care professionals and community organizations to improve the health of populations.

Resources Available for Patients/Families

Nurses need to be aware of a variety of resources that are available to patients and their families to provide comprehensive care. Some of these resources include:

- Community resources, such as home health agencies, meal delivery services and transportation services
- Support groups for patients and families dealing with specific conditions or illnesses
- Financial assistance programs for patients and families who may be struggling to pay health care costs
- Patient education materials and information on self-managing chronic conditions
- Caregiver support programs and respite care services
- Advance care planning resources and end-of-life care options

- Referrals to specialists or other health care providers as needed

An example of a resource that a nurse might need to know about for patient/family care is a local hospice program. Hospice programs provide care and support for patients and their families during the end-of-life process. Services may include symptom management, emotional and spiritual support and respite care for family members. The nurse will need to know how to refer patients and families to the hospice program and how to work with the hospice team to provide coordinated care.

Health Information to Meet Patient Needs

Health information is a crucial resource that nurses must know how to access and utilize in order to meet patient needs. This includes information on:

- **Diagnosis and treatment options** – Nurses need to understand the patient's diagnosis, potential complications and how to manage them, as well as any treatment options that are available.
- **Medications** – Nurses need to be familiar with the patient's medication regimen, including the name, dose, frequency and potential side effects of each medication.
- **Patient education** – Nurses need to provide patients with accurate and understandable information about their health condition, treatments and self-care.
- **Evidence-based practice** – Nurses need to be able to access and evaluate the latest research and guidelines to inform their practice and make evidence-based decisions about patient care.
- **Patient safety** – Nurses need to be aware of potential safety hazards and risks associated with the patient's condition and treatments and take appropriate measures to minimize these risks.

To meet these needs, nurses can access electronic health records, clinical databases and professional guidelines and journals. Patient education materials and other resources can also be used to provide patients and families with reliable health information.

Palliative/End-of-Life Care

Palliative or End-of-Life Patient/Caregiver Resources

Palliative care is a specialized form of medical treatment that aims to alleviate symptoms and improve the quality of life for patients living with serious, advanced or terminal illnesses. It focuses on managing pain and other symptoms rather than trying to cure the underlying condition.

Goals of Palliative Care

Table 20. Adapted from the WHO's Definition of Palliative Care

Goal	Description
Provide symptom relief	Palliative care aims to alleviate symptoms, such as pain, nausea and fatigue, to improve the patient's quality of life.
Normalize the dying process	Palliative care recognizes that dying is a normal part of life and seeks to provide comfort and support during this time.
Affirm life	Palliative care does not hasten or postpone death but rather affirms the patient's life and the importance of the person's experiences and relationships.
Support holistic care	Palliative care addresses the patient's and family's physical, emotional, social and spiritual needs to enhance the patient's quality of life.
Encourage active living	Palliative care aims to help patients live as actively as possible until death by providing support with activities of daily living and maintaining independence and dignity.
Support families	Palliative care also provides support to the patient's family during the patient's illness and in their own bereavement through counseling and grief support.

Palliative and end-of-life care can include a variety of resources to support patients and caregivers. Some examples include:

Hospice care – Hospice is not just a physical location but rather a concept of care that prioritizes compassion, concern and support for individuals nearing the end of their lives. Its main goal is to provide comfort and quality of life for those with terminal illnesses, focusing on symptom management, advance care planning, spiritual support and family assistance. It is important to note that hospice care is different from palliative care in that the latter allows for both curative and palliative treatments, while hospice care is provided when curative treatments are no longer being pursued.

Spiritual support – Many individuals find comfort in their spiritual or religious beliefs during the end-of-life process. This can include chaplain services, which provide spiritual counseling or access to religious or spiritual leaders.

Cultural support – End-of-life care should take into account the individual's cultural background. This can include providing access to traditional healers or cultural practices or respecting dietary restrictions or other cultural needs.

Physical support – End-of-life care should also include physical support, such as pain management, symptom control and assistance with activities of daily living. Occupational, physical or speech therapy can also be provided.

Support groups – Many patients and caregivers find comfort and support in talking with others who have had similar experiences. Support groups can provide emotional support and help people cope with end-of-life issues.

Online resources – There are many online resources, like websites and support groups, where patients and caregivers can find information and support.

End-of-Life Preferences

End-of-life preferences refer to the decisions and wishes individuals make regarding their medical treatment and care toward the end of their life.

These can encompass a wide range of options, including:

- Selecting or declining certain life-sustaining treatments, such as mechanical ventilation or dialysis
- Deciding where they would like to receive care, such as at home, in hospice or in a hospital
- Determining the level of pain management they desire
- Expressing the level of involvement they would like family members and loved ones to have in their care
- Outlining their preferences for medical treatment through advance directives, such as a living will, in case they become unable to communicate or make decisions for themselves
- Specifying their code status, also known as Do Not Resuscitate (DNR) orders, which indicates whether or not they would like to receive cardiopulmonary resuscitation (CPR) in the event of cardiac or respiratory arrest
- Requesting spiritual and emotional support

Table 21. Common Documents Utilized in End-of-Life Care and Their Key Considerations

Document	Description	Special Considerations
Advance directive	A legally binding document that outlines individuals' preferences for medical treatment in the event that they become incapacitated and unable to communicate.	Must comply with state-specific guidelines and regulations.
Physician's directive	A written statement that specifies an individual's desire to forgo life-sustaining treatments in the event of a terminal illness or injury.	Indicates specific measures to be used or withheld.
Do Not Resuscitate (DNR) order	A physician-issued directive that instructs health care providers to refrain from performing CPR in the event of cardiac or respiratory arrest. This order, also known as a DNR, is often requested by the patient's family and must be signed by a physician to be considered valid.	Often requested by the patient's family and must be signed by a physician to be valid.
Health care power of attorney	A document that designates a trusted individual to make health care decisions on patients' behalf in the event they become incapacitated.	May also be referred to as a medical power of attorney or health care proxy. Indicates specific measures to be used or withheld.

| Living will | A document that outlines individuals' preferences for medical treatment and end-of-life care in the event they become incapacitated and unable to communicate. | Must clearly identify specific treatments the individual wishes to receive or decline. |

Postmortem Care

After the patient has passed away, a nurse must prepare or delegate the preparation of the body for immediate viewing by the family, taking into consideration cultural customs and adhering to state laws and agency policies and procedures. In some cultures and circumstances, it may be important to allow the family to prepare or assist in preparing the body.

The body is prepared by closing the patient's eyes, replacing dentures, washing the body as needed and removing tubes and dressings. The body is positioned in a straight posture, leaving the pillow to support the head and prevent the pooling of blood and discoloration of the face.

Always provide the family with privacy and as much time as they need with the deceased person. In case of an unexpected or unanticipated death, the preparation of the body for viewing or release to a funeral home is guided by state laws and agency policies and procedures.

Organ Donation Process

Organ donation is an option for individuals who are legally competent. This can include any body part or the entire body. A person can make the decision to donate organs or provide anatomic gifts before death, or their immediate family can make the decision after death. Obtaining family permission at the time of donation is crucial.

Some individuals choose to carry donor cards, and some states allow individuals to indicate their willingness to donate on their driver's licenses. The agency responsible for coordinating organ donation can vary by state and community and may be referred to as an organ bank, organ-sharing network or organ-sharing alliance.

Organ and tissue donation is a complex process that requires adherence to specific legal guidelines and facility policies. This ensures that the donation is made in a lawful and ethical manner. One important step in this process is the immediate notification of the physician when organ donation is intended, as some tissues must be used within hours after death to be viable for transplantation. This timely notification allows for the proper handling and preservation of the donated organs and tissues, and it also ensures that the donation is made in a way that respects the wishes of the individual and the family.

Table 22. Steps of the Organ Donation Process

Step	Description
1	Identify potential organ donors.
2	Verify brain death.
3	Notify organ procurement organization.
4	Medical evaluation
5	Contact potential transplant recipients.
6	Transplantation surgery
7	Follow-up care
8	Legal and ethical considerations

This table provides an overview of the main steps in the organ donation process, but note that the actual process can be complex and may involve additional steps.

Regulatory Requirements for Reporting Death

In general, there are certain steps that must be followed in order to legally and properly report a death. Some of the common regulatory requirements for reporting death include:

1. **Notification of the next of kin** – The deceased's next of kin must be notified of the death as soon as possible.
2. **Obtaining a death certificate** – A death certificate must be obtained and completed by a physician or coroner. This document includes information, such as the cause of death, time of death and the deceased's personal details.
3. **Notifying authorities** – The death must be reported to the appropriate authorities, such as the local police or coroner's office.
4. **Obtaining a burial or cremation permit** – A permit must be obtained to bury or cremate the deceased. This permit is usually issued by the local

government and may require additional documentation, such as a death certificate.

5. **Registering the death** – The death must be registered with the local government and the relevant authorities. This may involve submitting a copy of the death certificate and other relevant documents.

6. **Legal and ethical considerations** – Legal and ethical considerations must be followed throughout the process.

Chapter 4: Elements of Interprofessional Care

Nursing Process/Clinical Judgment Measurement Model

Nursing Process

This topic is previously referenced in the book, but let's delve deeper into this topic to provide a more thorough understanding.

Table 23. Nursing Process

Step	Description
1. Assessment	Perform a comprehensive nursing assessment of the patient to gather data about physical, psychological, social and spiritual needs. Identify the patient's strengths, weaknesses and areas of concern.
2. Diagnosis	Make nursing diagnoses based on the data gathered during the assessment process. A nursing diagnosis is a statement that describes the patient's health status and identifies the patient's problems or needs.
3. Planning	Formulate and write outcome/goal statements and determine appropriate nursing interventions based on the patient's reality and evidence (research). Identify the patient's goals and expected outcomes, as well as the steps that will be taken to achieve them.
4. Implementation	Implement the care plan by delivering care to the patient. This includes administering medications, providing treatments and performing procedures.
5. Evaluation	Evaluate the outcomes and the nursing care that has been implemented. Determine if the patient's goals have been met, if the care plan was effective and if any changes or revisions are needed.

Step 1 – Assessment

During the assessment phase, the nurse's main focus is to gather as much information as possible about the patient's health status and needs. The first step is to complete a thorough health and medical history. This includes gathering information about the patient's past and present medical conditions, medications, allergies and family history.

The nurse should elicit as much information as possible during the assessment phase. One effective way is using open-ended questions instead of closed-ended questions that can be answered with a simple "yes" or "no." This approach allows patients to provide detailed information about their health and well-being, rather than limiting their responses to a single word.

Open-ended questions are particularly useful in this regard, as they encourage patients to provide more information about their situation. The following open-ended questions, suggested by Lusk & Fater (2013), are useful in screening for depression in older patients:

• What made you come here today?

• What do you think your problem is?

• What do you think caused your problem?

• Are you worried about anything in particular?

• What have you tried to do about the problem so far?

• What would you like me to do about your problem?

• Is there anything else you would like to discuss today?

In addition to obtaining information verbally from the patient, nurses also gather information by performing a physical assessment, taking vital signs and noting diagnostic test results. This information is considered objective information.

Both the subjective and objective information obtained during the assessment phase are used to identify the patient's strengths, weaknesses and areas of concern and to make appropriate nursing diagnoses, formulate outcome/goal statements, determine appropriate nursing interventions and evaluate the patient's progress.

Step 2 – Nursing Diagnosis

Clinical reasoning is the process of thoroughly analyzing information, recognizing cues, sorting and organizing the data and determining a patient's strengths and unmet needs in order to make an appropriate diagnosis.

A structured method known as the PES system can be used to succinctly identify a patient's needs and concerns. The PES system comprises three elements:

P (problem) – A brief nursing diagnosis label that represents a pattern of related cues sourced from the official NANDA-I list.

E (etiology) – The underlying cause or contributor to the problem, represented by the "related to" phrase or etiology.

S (symptoms) – The symptoms the nurse observes during the assessment are described as the defining characteristics phrase.

This system helps nurses organize and communicate their assessment findings in a clear and consistent manner.

The process of identifying patterns and symptoms can be broken down into the following steps:

A. Identify and highlight important symptoms (defining characteristics). As you review the patient's assessment information, ask yourself: Is this typical? Is this ideal? Is this a problem for the patient? You may also need to validate information with the patient.
B. Create a list of the symptoms you have identified and highlighted.
C. Cluster together similar symptoms.
D. Analyze and interpret the symptoms. What do these symptoms signify or represent when they occur together?
E. Using the NANDA-I list, a nurse can carefully select a suitable nursing diagnosis label that corresponds with the specific defining characteristics and nursing diagnosis definition of the patient's condition.

Step 3 – Planning

The planning phase includes the identification of priorities, as well as the determination of appropriate patient-specific outcomes and interventions.

When prioritizing nursing diagnoses, the patient's immediate needs should be considered first, using the ABC approach. Additionally, Maslow's hierarchy of needs should be taken into account, giving priority to problems that may be life-threatening. For example, a patient with asthma who is experiencing difficulty clearing their airway due to increased secretions and increased use of an inhaler would have a higher priority than a patient who is experiencing anxiety, which is considered a lower-level need in Maslow's hierarchy.

It is important for the nurse to record the care plan in detail, including the prioritized nursing diagnostic statements, desired outcomes and implemented interventions.

This documentation can be done either through electronic means or traditional pen-and-paper methods.

Step 4 – Implementation

The implementation phase involves executing the individualized, agreed-upon interventions in the care plan. These interventions often aim to manage symptoms rather than cure the underlying medical condition. The focus of nursing care is on providing support and assistance to patients and their families, helping them function at the highest level possible.

This is the stage where the nurse actually provides nursing care by carrying out the interventions that have been tailored to the patient's specific needs.

Step 5 – Evaluation

Evaluation is an ongoing aspect and is not limited to the end of the process. It involves reassessing patients and comparing their conditions before and after the interventions. The nurse's assessment of a patient's response to interventions is valuable in determining if adjustments need to be made to the care plan.

For example, if a patient is given medication to alleviate pain and the nurse observes that the patient is experiencing relief and no side effects, it suggests that the intervention was effective. The nurse's documentation of the patient's response is beneficial for the entire health care team. In addition to ongoing assessment, proper documentation is a vital aspect of the evaluation phase. The nurse should use the facility's designated documentation tool to record all nursing activities and the outcomes of the interventions.

Problem-oriented charting, which involves evaluating care and patient outcomes, is often used in many facilities. It is also essential to document all actions taken, as it serves as a legal requirement; if something is not recorded, it is considered as not done.

Keeping accurate and detailed records of nursing interventions and patient outcomes is crucial for providing quality care and protecting the facility and the nurse in case of a legal dispute.

Strategies to Individualize Care

Original, individualized care occurs when the nurse recognizes the patient as a unique individual and adapts nursing care to the patient's specific experiences, behaviors, feelings and perceptions, including the events associated with the person's illness, home life, work, physical indicators and preferred coping strategies.

There are several strategies that nurses can use to provide individualized care for patients. Some of these include:

1. **Building a therapeutic relationship** – Nurses should work to establish a relationship of trust and respect with their patients. This can involve actively listening to patients, responding to their concerns and providing emotional support.
2. **Assessing and identifying patient needs** – Nurses should conduct a thorough assessment of their patients' physical, emotional and social needs. This information can be used to develop an individualized care plan that addresses each patient's specific needs.
3. **Involving patients in their own care** – Nurses should encourage patients to participate in their own care by providing them with information and education about their condition, treatment options and self-care strategies.
4. **Using patient-centered communication** – Nurses should use language and communication techniques that are easy for patients to understand and that respect their cultural and personal values.
5. **Collaborating with other members of the health care team** – Nurses should work closely with other members of the health care team, such as physicians, social workers and physical therapists, to ensure that patients receive comprehensive and coordinated care.
6. **Continuously monitoring and evaluating the care** – Nurses should regularly evaluate the effectiveness of their individualized care plans and make adjustments as needed to ensure they are meeting their patients' needs.
7. **Incorporating a holistic approach** – Nursing care should address patients as a whole, including their physical, emotional, social and spiritual needs.
8. **Being flexible** – The care should be adaptable to patients' changing needs, allowing for modifications as the patients' conditions change.

Interprofessional Collaboration

Role within the Interdisciplinary Team

An interdisciplinary approach to care is the most effective way to meet patients' needs. This approach brings together different health care professionals with different areas of expertise to work together in a coordinated manner. By pooling their knowledge and skills, the health care team can provide comprehensive, holistic care that addresses the patient's physical, emotional and social needs.

Several studies have demonstrated the detrimental effects that poor communication between health care providers has on patient outcomes. For instance, studies have shown that a lack of communication between doctors and nurses can result in drug errors, treatment delays and other unfavorable events.

Nurse-Physician Collaboration

It is possible to promote nurse-physician collaboration in a number of ways. Setting up regular meetings between nurses and doctors to discuss patient care is one efficient strategy. This can include frequent communication opportunities, such as daily rounds, weekly team meetings or other events.

Open and straightforward communication is the key to nurse-physician partnership success. Doctors and nurses should feel at ease talking about patient care difficulties, exchanging information and seeking assistance when necessary. By doing so, it may be possible to avoid misconceptions and guarantee that patients get the best treatment possible.

Agree to talk about disagreements as they happen. The health care team can resolve issues, stop disagreements from worsening and prevent an adverse effect on patient care by dealing with disagreements promptly and professionally.

Collaboration with Other Members of the Health Care Team

Everyone needs to have a fundamental grasp of their roles and responsibilities in order to interact effectively with other health care professionals, such as social workers, dietitians and physical, occupational and respiratory therapists.

Reading pertinent articles and books is one approach to learning more about these jobs. This can give a broad overview of the duties held by various health care professionals and point out areas where cooperation might be especially helpful.

Speaking directly with individuals in these organizations is another efficient way to learn about these responsibilities. Asking questions, taking part in interdisciplinary case conferences or observing other health care professionals at work are all examples of how to achieve this.

Conferences on interdisciplinary cases are crucial to collaborative practice. These conferences give team members a chance to learn about the contributions different health care professionals make to patient care and might point out potential areas for fruitful collaboration. Such gatherings demonstrate a facility's dedication to teamwork.

Interprofessional Rounding

Interprofessional rounding is the process of gathering several health care experts, including doctors, nurses, social workers and other team members, on a frequent basis to talk about patient care. This can include frequent communication opportunities, such as daily rounds, weekly team meetings or other events.

The goal of interprofessional rounding is to improve the coordination of care, ensure that patients receive the most appropriate treatment and identify any potential issues before they become major problems.

During interprofessional rounding, team members discuss each patient's condition, treatment plan and any changes in their condition. This allows team members to share information and coordinate care, which can lead to improved patient outcomes. Additionally, it allows for the identification of potential issues such as medication errors, delays in treatment or other adverse events that can be addressed in a timely manner.

Care Coordination

Care coordination is recognized as a vital strategy by the Institute of Medicine to enhance the effectiveness, safety and efficiency of the American health care system. Providing targeted and well-designed care coordination to the right patients can improve outcomes for patients, health care providers and payers alike.

However, there are certain obstacles within the American health care system that need to be overcome to provide this type of care. It is crucial to redesign the health care system to improve care coordination for the following reasons:

1. The current health care system is often disjointed, with varying processes among primary care and specialty sites.
2. Many patients may not understand why they are being referred, how to schedule appointments or what steps to take after visiting a specialist. This lack of understanding can lead to confusion, frustration and a lack of trust in the health care system.
3. Specialists do not consistently receive clear reasons for referrals or enough information on previous tests, while primary care physicians do not receive information about what happened during a referral visit.
4. Referral staff often deal with multiple processes and lost information, leading to less efficient care.

In primary care practices, care coordination is of particular importance, as it helps ensure that patients receive high-quality, high-value health care. There are two main ways to achieve coordinated care: through broad approaches that are commonly used to improve health care delivery and through specific care coordination activities.

Examples of broad care coordination approaches include:

- Teamwork among health care providers
- Care management programs
- Medication management
- Health information technology
- A patient-centered medical home model

Specific actions such as:

- Identifying and assigning roles and responsibilities among health care providers
- Promoting open communication and sharing of information
- Facilitating smooth transitions of care
- Evaluating patient needs and objectives
- Planning ahead for potential issues
- Regularly assessing progress
- Encouraging patient autonomy and self-care
- Linking patients to community resources
- Ensuring the efficient utilization of available resources to match patient needs

Collaborative Problem-Solving

Collaborative problem-solving involves working with other health care professionals to identify and address issues related to patient care. This can include identifying potential problems, developing and implementing solutions and evaluating the effectiveness of those solutions.

One example of collaborative problem-solving for nurses might be addressing the issue of medication errors in a hospital setting. A team of nurses, doctors and pharmacy staff might come together to identify the root causes of medication errors, such as poor communication between health care providers or unclear labeling on medication. They would then develop and implement solutions, such as implementing a standardized communication protocol or redesigning the labeling system for medications.

Also, the team would set up a procedure for recording and assessing the success of these solutions, such as keeping track of the number of medication errors before and after the introduction of the new protocol or checking on staff adherence to the new labeling system.

Care Coordination and Transition Management

Community Resources

To enable them to give their patients the best care possible outside the hospital, nurses working in community settings may need to be conversant with a range of local services. Some examples of these resources are:

- **Community health clinics** – Anyone in the community can receive primary care at these clinics in addition to additional medical services, like immunizations and screenings, regardless of their financial situation.
- **Home health agencies** – For patients who are aged, incapacitated or recovering from an illness or surgery, these agencies offer nursing, therapy and other health care services in the comfort of their own homes.
- **Support groups** – There are many various kinds of support groups available for patients, including those for persons with a particular ailment or disease and those facing a particular obstacle in life; there are also groups for caregivers.
- **Social services** – For patients who are struggling with poverty or other socioeconomic determinants of health, social service organizations in many communities can offer help with things like housing, food and transportation.
- **Public health departments** – In addition to tools for patient education and vaccination programs, public health departments can give nurses information about public health problems and epidemics.
- **Community centers** – Community centers frequently offer a variety of services to the general public, including health screenings, exercise classes and educational initiatives, which can be helpful for patients trying to enhance their general health and well-being.

Interdisciplinary Collaboration Integration Methods

Discharge Planning

The smooth transition of patients from one level of care to the next is made possible through discharge planning. It entails developing a specialized plan that gives patients specific instructions and direction as they transition from the hospital to their homes or long-term care facilities. Effective discharge planning aims to enhance the patient's overall quality of life by preserving continuity of care and lowering the possibility of unanticipated difficulties or readmissions. Discharge planning is necessary for hospitals to maintain accreditation in the United States.

Effective discharge planning necessitates the participation of an interdisciplinary team, and collaboration is a key element. The team, under the direction of the doctor, is responsible for determining if the patient is ready for discharge, developing a unique discharge plan and conveying it to the discharge nurse or other designated people.

It is important to have a thorough discharge plan, but it is also crucial to make sure it is successfully conveyed to the patient, all required providers and other parties.

Mobility

Getting in and out of bed, walking and climbing stairs are just a few of the basic functional movements that a medical-surgical nurse will assess regarding a patient's mobility. Any physical restrictions or ailments—such as muscle weakness, joint pain or a recent operation—that may limit the patient's movement should be taken into consideration during the examination. The nurse will develop a strategy for helping the patient regain or maintain mobility based on the assessment. This plan might include physical therapy, exercises and the use of assistive devices. The nurse will also keep an eye on the patient's development and modify the strategy as necessary.

There are several guidelines and tools that medical professionals can use to assess a patient's mobility. Some commonly used tools are:

1. **The Timed Up and Go (TUG) test** – This examination gauges a patient's capacity for standing up from a seated position, moving a short distance and then sitting down again. It is frequently employed to determine a patient's risk of falling.
2. **The Five Times Sit to Stand (FTSST) test** – This examination gauges a patient's capacity for standing from a seated posture and then sitting down once more. It is frequently utilized to evaluate lower body muscle function and strength.
3. **The Berg Balance Scale (BBS)** – This examination gauges a patient's stability, balance and capacity for carrying out practical tasks, including reaching, turning and stepping.
4. **The Barthel Index of Activities of Daily Living** – This examination gauges a patient's capacity for carrying out fundamental, everyday tasks, like showering, dressing and using the restroom.
5. **The Functional Reach Test** – This test measures a patient's ability to reach forward while maintaining balance.

Mobility can be graded on a scale to indicate the level of difficulty a person may have with movement. The most common scale used is the Functional Mobility Scale (FMS), which grades mobility on a scale of 0 to 4.

Table 24. FMS Grading of Mobility

Grade	Description
0	The patient is unable to move and requires full assistance.
1	The patient is able to move but requires significant assistance.
2	The patient is able to move but requires moderate assistance.
3	The patient is able to move with minimal assistance.
4	The patient is able to move independently.

Physical Therapy

When it comes to helping patients who struggle with mobility challenges regain their independence, physical therapy plays an essential role. For a patient who has recently undergone hip replacement surgery, for instance, physical therapy would be an essential part of the rehabilitation and recovery process.

The physical therapist will begin by conducting a thorough examination of the patient in order to determine the present degree of mobility, strength, flexibility and function. In addition to this, the physical therapist will take into account the patient's level of pain, any other physical limitations and the patient's desired outcomes regarding recovery.

Based on the evaluation, the physical therapist will develop an individualized treatment plan to help the patient regain mobility. This plan may include:

- Exercises to improve the patient's strength, flexibility and range of motion in the hip and leg
- Gait training to help the patient learn how to walk safely and efficiently with the new hip
- Techniques to manage pain and reduce inflammation
- Education on proper posture and body mechanics to minimize stress on the hip
- The use of assistive devices, such as crutches, canes or walkers
- Balance and coordination exercises to improve the patient's stability and reduce the risk of falls

The physical therapist will also educate the patient and family on how to properly perform exercises and care for the hip at home. The therapist will work closely with the patient's surgeon and other members of the health care team to ensure that the patient receives comprehensive and coordinated care.

Physical therapy sessions will typically be scheduled on a regular basis, such as two to three times a week until the patient's goals are met and the individual is able to move around independently. The therapist will monitor the patient's progress and make any necessary adjustments to the treatment plan.

Health History Assessment from Multiple Sources

When conducting a health history assessment, nurses typically begin by talking with the patient and asking about medical history, current symptoms and any medications or supplements the person is taking. This information can help the nurse identify any risk factors or underlying conditions that may impact the patient's care.

In addition to obtaining information from the patient, nurses also often review medical records, laboratory results and other relevant documentation from other health care providers. This can provide a more complete picture of the patient's health history, including any previous diagnoses, treatments or procedures. Medication lists should also be reviewed, as they can help the nurse identify any potential drug interactions or side effects that may impact the patient's care.

Family members or caregivers can provide valuable insights into the patient's health history too, including information about inherited medical conditions, previous treatments and any changes in the patient's health or behavior.

Discharge Procedures

Table 25. Discharge Procedure

Steps	Description
1	Before the day of discharge, notify the patient and the designated family or caregivers of the anticipated discharge date and time.
2	Obtain a written discharge order from the treating physician, including any specific instructions for post-discharge care. If the patient chooses to leave against medical advice, ensure that the necessary paperwork and consent forms are completed.

3	If the patient requires ongoing medical care or assistance upon discharge, make sure that appropriate arrangements have been made with the relevant home care agency or community health facility.
4	Prior to discharge, review and discuss the patient's individualized discharge care plan, which includes any updates made during their hospital stay, with the patient and the family or designated caregivers. Ensure that they understand the plan and any instructions for post-discharge care.
5	Create a comprehensive medication list for the patient, including drug name, dosage, frequency and any potential side effects or interactions. Review this list with the patient and their family or designated caregivers and ensure that the medication schedule aligns with the patient's daily routine and lifestyle to promote compliance and prevent any improper administration.
6	Review any self-care procedures or treatments that the patient or the family will need to perform at home, such as wound care or administering medication. Provide hands-on demonstrations and written instructions and follow up to ensure that the patient and the family understand the procedures and are able to perform them correctly.
7	If necessary, provide specific dietary and activity instructions to the patient and the family or designated caregivers and explain the reasons behind them. Include these instructions in the patient's discharge instruction sheet.
8	Confirm with the physician if the patient has a follow-up appointment scheduled and communicate the date, time and location to the patient if necessary.
9	Retrieve any personal belongings or valuables that the patient had left in the facility's safe and review each item with the patient to ensure that nothing is missing. Obtain the patient's signature on a document verifying receipt of the valuables.
10	Retrieve any medications the patient brought and have a pharmacist check them to ensure they are safe to take and not expired or contaminated.

11	Perform a final check of the patient's vital signs, as appropriate and record them on the discharge summary form. If any signs are abnormal or outside the expected range, notify the physician immediately.
12	Assist the patient with getting dressed, if necessary, and ensure the person is comfortable before leaving the facility.
13	Collect the patient's personal belongings from the room, ensuring that nothing is left behind or misplaced.
14	Before the patient leaves the facility, conduct a final check of the room to ensure all personal belongings have been collected and nothing is left behind. Help the patient into a wheelchair or onto a stretcher, if needed, and escort them to the exit. Provide any necessary assistance for patients leaving by ambulance.
15	After the patient has exited the facility, strip the bed linens and notify the housekeeping staff that the room is ready for final cleaning.

Patient/Family-Centered Care

Patient- and family-centered care is a holistic and person-centered approach to health care that values the unique needs, preferences and perspectives of patients and their families. It emphasizes collaboration and partnership between health care providers, patients and families throughout the health care process. This approach aims to empower patients and families to actively participate in their own care and decision-making and address their emotional and psychological needs.

The following are core concepts of patient- and family-centered care:

1. **Respect and dignity** – This approach values the unique needs, perspectives and experiences of patients and their families. Health care practitioners listen to and honor patient and family perspectives and choices.
2. **Information-sharing** – Clear, complete and unbiased information is provided to patients and families in a way that is easy to understand so that they can make informed decisions about their care.
3. **Participation** – Patients and families are encouraged and empowered to take an active role in their care and are supported in making decisions about their treatment at the level they choose.
4. **Collaboration** – Patient- and family-centered care promotes a culture of teamwork, where patients, families, health care practitioners and leaders work

together in all aspects of health care, including policy, program development, facility design, professional education, research and care delivery.

Care Coordination and Transition

Care coordination involves organizing patient care activities among multiple participants to facilitate the delivery of health services. It is the process of ensuring that the patient's needs are met throughout the entirety of the care process. This is accomplished by identifying potential barriers to continuity of care, communicating with other health care providers and agencies and facilitating the transfer of patient information.

Patients are said to be transitioning from one level of care or environment to another during the process known as "care transitions." Moves from the hospital to the patient's home, from the emergency department to inpatient care, or from one health care facility to another are all examples of transitions that fall under this category. It is also possible for care transitions to take place inside the same physical site, such as when a patient is moved from the intensive care unit to the regular medical-surgical unit.

It is necessary to make sure that the transition from one type of treatment to another is as easy and unnoticeable for patients as possible in order to accomplish good care coordination.

Planning things out thoroughly is the first step toward achieving efficient care coordination. This comprises the adoption of automated workflows, real-time transition data and a clear communication road across providers, including primary care and subspecialists, as well as employees. In addition, this includes a clear communication pathway between patients and staff.

The coordination process can be streamlined with the use of automated workflows, which makes it both more efficient and accurate. The timely exchange of patient information is essential to guaranteeing continuity of care; real-time transition data makes it possible to share patient information at the appropriate time. To ensure that all stakeholders are informed and participating in the care process, there must be a transparent communication pathway between the various providers and workers.

In summary, care coordination and transition include:

- Determining the patient's requirements and locating any potential obstacles to maintaining the continuity of treatment
- Coordinating the patient's treatment with the help of other medical professionals and organizations through communication and collaboration

- Ensuring that transferred patient information is accurate and comprehensive while simultaneously facilitating its transfer
- Helping the patient and the family comprehend the treatment plan and the subsequent steps in the process
- Keeping track of the patient's development and modifying the treatment strategy accordingly as new information emerges
- Making sure that the patient's requirements are being fulfilled after a care transition by following up with the patient and any other health care providers who were involved in the patient's care.

Interprofessional Roles and Responsibilities

Interprofessional duties and responsibilities are the numerous tasks and functions that are performed by multiple health care experts in collaboration with one another to offer comprehensive patient care. This type of care is provided by a team of health care professionals. Tasks such as diagnosis, treatment planning, patient education and ongoing care coordination are some examples of the roles and responsibilities that are distributed among the various medical specialties, such as physicians, nurses, pharmacists and therapists. These roles and responsibilities also include coordinating ongoing care.

1. A team of medical professionals, including doctors and nurses, collaborates in a hospital setting to diagnose and treat patients. The initial diagnosis and the formulation of a treatment plan may fall under the purview of the attending physician, while the nurse may be accountable for administering medication, monitoring vital signs and providing patient education.
2. Pharmacists and physicians work together to ensure patients receive the correct pharmaceutical regimen for their conditions. The physician may be the one to make the final decision on the prescription that is appropriate for the patient, despite the fact that the pharmacist may analyze the patient's medication history and give recommendations to the physician.
3. Patients are assisted in their recovery from injuries or diseases by a collaborative effort between physical therapists and occupational therapists. It is possible that the physical therapist's primary focus will be enhancing the patient's physical strength and mobility, while the occupational therapist's primary focus will be helping the patient regain their capacity to carry out day-to-day tasks.
4. Collaboration between social workers and case managers helps to provide coordinated care for patients with many complex demands. While the social worker may offer patients emotional support and connect them with community resources, the case manager's primary responsibility is to coordinate the patient's

services and ensure that care is consistent throughout all the health care venues in which the person receives treatment.

5. An interdisciplinary team of health care professionals, including a nutritionist, pharmacist, nurse and physician, work together to manage a patient who has diabetes, to provide comprehensive care, including monitoring blood sugar levels, adjusting medication, discussing diet and physical activity and providing education to the patient.

Continuum of Care

A patient is said to get a coordinated and all-encompassing set of health care treatments known as a continuum of care over the course of treatment. It includes the management of acute care, rehabilitation and ongoing treatment of chronic illnesses in addition to disease prevention and early intervention. The provision of treatment that is coordinated and effective and satisfies the patient's requirements at every point throughout the course of the person's health journey is the objective of a continuum of care.

Examples of the different levels of care within a continuum of care include:

1. **Prevention and wellness** – Activities such as health education, screenings and vaccines are included in this level of care. These kinds of activities prevent sickness and enhance general health and well-being.
2. **Primary care** – The patient's primary care physician or nurse practitioner delivers this level of care, which consists of routine check-ups, screenings and the management of common ailments.
3. **Acute care** – The diagnosis and treatment of serious injuries or illnesses are the primary focus of this level of care, which is administered in a hospital setting.
4. **Rehabilitation** – Services such as physical therapy, occupational therapy and speech therapy are included in this level of treatment, which is primarily geared toward assisting patients in their recovery from disease or injury.
5. **Long-term care** – Patients who have chronic diseases that require continuing monitoring and support receive this level of care. Patients who require this level of care have complex medical needs. This level of care encompasses a wide range of services, including those provided in the home, nursing homes and assisted living communities.
6. **End-of-life care** – Patients who are nearing the end of their lives receive this level of care, which focuses on making them as comfortable as possible and offering them support. This level of care consists of hospice care, palliative care and assistance for family members going through bereavement.

The Role of Medical-Surgical Nurses

Patients who are scheduled to have surgery are in good hands with medical-surgical nurses because they are a key element of the continuum of care. They are essential in the process of delivering care before, during and after surgical procedures.

During the preoperative phase, medical-surgical nurses collaborate with patients to educate them about the upcoming procedure, evaluate their medical history and present condition and ensure that patients are adequately prepared for the operation. In addition to this, they collaborate with the surgical team to examine the patient's medical history and make certain all the required equipment and supplies are in the operating room.

During the surgical procedure, it is the medical-surgical nurses' job to keep an eye on the patient's vital signs and offer assistance to the other members of the surgical team. They also help with placing the patient, giving medication and getting the patient ready to be transported to the recovery room.

The postoperative phase is an important time for medical-surgical nurses since they are responsible for monitoring the patient's condition and giving care to aid in their recovery. They are responsible for managing the patient's pain, administering medication, monitoring the patient's vital signs, educating the patient and the family members and providing emotional support. In addition, they coordinate their efforts with the other members of the patient's health care team in order to check if the patient is making the expected progress and make any required revisions to the treatment plan.

Patients at Risk for Readmissions

Patients who have chronic conditions—such as heart failure, chronic obstructive pulmonary disease (COPD) and diabetes—as well as patients who have recently undergone a surgical procedure or been discharged from the intensive care unit are at an increased risk for readmission to the hospital.

Inadequate follow-up care after release, a lack of social support and poor communication between health care professionals are some other variables that can raise the risk of readmission for a patient.

Quality Patient Outcome Measures

The Donabedian model, named after the physician and researcher who formulated it, is a widely recognized framework for assessing and comparing the quality of health care organizations. The model classifies measures used to evaluate quality into three distinct categories: structure, process and outcome.

Structural measures provide a comprehensive overview of a health care provider's capacity to deliver high-quality care. These measures take into account the systems and processes the organization puts in place to ensure the best possible outcomes for patients. One example of a structural measure is the utilization of electronic health records (EHRs) or medication order entry systems.

Another structural measure is the proportion of board-certified physicians within an organization. Board certification is an indicator of a physician's expertise and commitment to ongoing professional development. A higher proportion of board-certified physicians suggests that an organization is staffed by highly qualified and skilled professionals. Finally, the ratio of providers to patients is another structural measure that can be used to evaluate a health care provider's capacity. A lower ratio may indicate that the organization is stretched thin and may be unable to provide timely and comprehensive care.

For evaluating the level of care that a health care practitioner gives patients, **process measures** are an extremely useful instrument. These measurements provide an idea of the steps an organization takes to ensure and improve the health of patients, and they are reflective of guidelines that are generally accepted for clinical practice. Process measures include things like the percentage of patients who get cancer screenings or immunizations, for instance. Another example is the number of patients who get their blood pressure checked. This metric can shed insight into the degree to which the health care professional places a greater emphasis on preventing sickness and encouraging overall wellness as opposed to merely treating already existing issues.

This metric can be used to determine how effectively the health care professional manages the treatment of patients who have chronic diseases. Patients can be informed by these process measurements of the type of care they can anticipate receiving for a given ailment or illness, and these measures can also contribute to an improvement in the health outcomes that are achieved. It is important to point out that the vast majority of the quality metrics utilized for public reporting in the health care industry are process measurements.

Outcome measures analyze how the provision of medical services or the performance of interventions affects the patients' overall health. These indicators offer comprehension of how successfully the health care service or intervention improves patient outcomes. The following are some examples of measures of outcomes:

- The risk of death experienced by patients as a result of undergoing a surgical procedure
- The number of patients who suffer from problems or illnesses during their time in the hospital

However, it is essential to keep in mind that outcomes are the product of a variety of factors, many of which are not necessarily within the health care provider's control. Despite the fact that outcome measures may appear to be the ultimate benchmark for measuring quality, it is important to keep in mind that outcomes are the result of a variety of factors. Methods of risk adjustment, such as mathematical models, are utilized in order to take these aspects into consideration and account for the variations that exist within a population.

Documentation

Documentation of Patient Care

In order to effectively communicate with other members of the health care team and provide information for professionals involved in accreditation, credentialing, legal, regulatory, reimbursement, research and quality activities, RNs are required to document their work and the outcomes of their work. This documentation guarantees that patients receive continuous treatment, supports the reimbursement of providers for their services and enables continuous attempts to improve quality.

It is imperative that nursing documentation is of high quality in order to guarantee efficient communication and care continuity across all members of the health care team. The following qualities and characteristics should be exhibited by documentation:

- **Accessibility** – Ensure that all members of the health care team, as well as those involved in accreditation, credentialing, legal, regulatory, reimbursement, research and quality operations, have easy access to documentation; it should be easily searchable.
- **Accuracy, relevance and consistency** – It needs to be correct, pertinent to patients' health and the care they are receiving and consistent with all the other documents.
- **Auditability** – Auditing should be possible in order to guarantee that the documentation is accurate and comprehensive.
- **Clarity, conciseness and completeness** – Documentation should be clear, concise and complete, providing all the necessary information about the patient's condition and care.
- **Thoughtful** – Documentation should reflect thoughtful consideration of the patient's condition and care.
- **Timeliness** – Documentation should be contemporaneous with the patient's care and sequential in order to provide a complete picture of the patient's condition and care.

- **Retrievable** – Documentation should be retrievable on a permanent basis in a nursing-specific manner.
- **Readability** – Documentation must be optimized for readability and legibility, regardless of the device it is viewed on. This means the resolution and related qualities of EHR content should be carefully considered so the documentation is easily readable and understandable on all devices, including computers, tablets and smartphones.

Electronic Health Records

EHRs are digital versions of traditional paper medical records. They contain a patient's medical history, including demographic information, vital signs, medications, allergies, immunizations, laboratory test results and other relevant health information. EHRs enable health care providers to access a patient's complete medical history in real time, which can improve patient care, reduce medical errors and increase efficiency and cost-effectiveness. They also allow for easy sharing of information between health care providers, which improves continuity of care and can facilitate care coordination.

Downtime Procedures

Downtime procedures refer to the steps that health care organizations take to ensure continuity of care during system outages or other disruptions. These procedures help minimize the impact of such disruptions on patient care and can include steps such as:

- **Establishing a backup plan** – Having a plan in place for how to handle system outages, including identifying critical systems and prioritizing which functions need to be restored first
- **Training staff** – Ensuring that staff is trained on the backup plan and knows what to do in the event of a disruption
- **Establishing communication protocols** – Establishing protocols for how staff will communicate during an outage, including who to contact and how to reach them
- **Identifying critical patient populations** – Identifying patients who are most likely to be affected by an outage and developing plans to ensure their care is not disrupted
- **Testing the plan** – Regularly testing the backup plan to ensure it is effective and identify any areas that need improvement
- **Keeping paper records** – Having paper records as a backup in case electronic systems are unavailable
- **Documenting the incident** – Documenting the incident and analyzing the cause of the outage and what can be done to prevent it from happening again in the future

Coaching for Documentation Performance Improvement

Implementing downtime procedures can help minimize the impact of system outages on patient care and ensure that continuity of care is maintained.

Coaching for documentation performance improvement is a process of providing guidance and support to nurses and other health care professionals to help them improve their documentation practices. This can include providing training on documentation best practices, as well as working one-on-one with staff to identify and address specific documentation issues. The goal of coaching is to help improve the quality and completeness of documentation, which can lead to better communication, continuity of care and overall patient outcomes.

Some common coaching activities are:

- Providing training and education on documentation best practices and standards
- Reviewing documentation with staff to identify areas for improvement and provide feedback
- Providing guidance on how to document patient care in a clear, concise and accurate manner
- Offering support and resources to help staff understand and comply with regulatory requirements related to documentation
- Helping staff understand the importance of documentation in the patients' overall care
- Assessing the effectiveness of the coaching and modifying the approach as necessary

Technology

Technology, Equipment Use and Troubleshooting

The utilization of technology and equipment, as well as the ability to troubleshoot, are essential components of nursing documentation. When documenting patient care, nurses and other medical professionals use a wide variety of technologies and pieces of specialized equipment. Some examples of this technology and equipment include EHRs, medical devices and other specialized tools.

Technology and equipment use:

- Training should be provided to nurses and other health care professionals on the correct use of technology and equipment, including instruction on how to document patient care using EHRs and other forms of technology.
- It is essential for the personnel to have a thorough understanding of the technology and the equipment that they are utilizing, including the navigation of the system, the entry of data and the retrieval of information.
- They should also be knowledgeable about the capabilities and features of the technology and equipment, as well as how to use those features and capabilities to document patient care in a way that is clear, succinct and accurate.

Troubleshooting:

- Training on how to troubleshoot typical issues that may develop with technology and equipment should be provided to nurses and other people working in the health care industry.
- They should be knowledgeable about the techniques for troubleshooting the technology and equipment that they are employing in their work.
- Moreover, they should be aware of the contact information for technical support and know how to get assistance when it is required.

Technology Trends in Health Care

The landscape of health care is being rapidly transformed as a result of technological advancements and there are a number of trends that are now impacting the business. The following are some examples of recent technological advances in the health care industry:

1. **EHRs** – Because they allow for better communication, continuity of care and reduced medical errors, EHRs are gaining popularity. This is due to the fact that they enable real-time access to patient information.
2. **Telehealth** – Telemedicine, teleconsultations and remote patient monitoring are all examples of telehealth services, which refers to the use of technology to deliver health care services to patients remotely. Patients are therefore able to receive medical care without physically going to a health care center.
3. **Artificial intelligence (AI)** – In the medical field, AI is being used to enhance the precision and timeliness of diagnoses, as well as to facilitate decision-making and automate mundane chores.
4. **Wearable technology** – Wearable technology—such as smartwatches, fitness trackers and other gadgets—can assist in the monitoring of patients' vital signs and other data linked to their health, which in turn enables health care providers to spot potential health issues at an earlier stage.

5. **Internet of Things (IoT)** – Connecting medical equipment through the IoT enables the collection and analysis of real-time patient data, which in turn enables health care providers to make decisions that are more informed about their patients.
6. **Robotics** – In the medical field, robots are increasingly being utilized to carry out procedures like operations and to help provide care to patients, including rehabilitation and physical therapy.

Nursing Informatics

The field of nursing informatics is a blend of nursing science, computer science and information science. Its primary focus is on the application of technology and information in order to enhance the quality of care provided to patients. The following categories are included in the scope of the field of nursing informatics:

1. **EHRs and other health information systems** – Nursing informatics professionals work to ensure that EHRs and other health information systems are user-friendly and efficient and that they support the documentation and management of patient care.
2. **Data analysis and decision-making** – Nursing informatics professionals analyze data from EHRs and other health information systems to identify patterns and trends and use this information to make evidence-based decisions about patient care.
3. **Education and training** – Nursing informatics professionals educate and train nurses and other health care professionals on the use of technology and information systems in patient care.
4. **Research** – Nursing informatics professionals conduct research on the use of technology and information systems in patient care, including the impact on patient outcomes and the effectiveness of various technologies and systems.
5. **Standards and regulations** – Nursing informatics professionals work to ensure that the use of technology and information systems in patient care complies with relevant standards and regulations.

Chapter 5: Professional Concepts

Communication

Chain of Command

The chain of command in nursing refers to the hierarchy of leadership and authority within the nursing profession. It establishes a clear line of communication and accountability, ensuring that decisions are made at the appropriate level and that everyone knows who to report to and who to contact if they have any issues or concerns.

The chain of command in nursing typically starts with entry-level positions, such as nurse technicians and staff nurses, who are responsible for providing direct patient care. It then progresses to higher-level positions, such as charge nurses, nursing managers and directors, who are responsible for supervising staff and managing specific units or departments. The highest level of nursing leadership is the chief nursing officer (CNO), who is responsible for overall nursing strategy and decision-making within the organization. In some cases, the CNO may report to the facility's president or CEO.

Communication Skills

In nursing, effective communication is a fundamental aspect of providing quality care to patients. Nurses must possess the ability to communicate clearly, confidently and in a manner that is easily understandable to patients, families, physicians and other health care staff. This includes explaining medical concepts, treatments and procedures, as well as providing regular updates on patients' conditions.

Active Listening

Active listening is a vital communication skill for nurses that involves actively paying attention to what others are saying, understanding their message and providing an appropriate response. By using active listening techniques, nurses can better understand patients' needs and experiences, leading to improved patient outcomes.

Some active listening techniques that nurses can use include:

1. **Observing the speaker's behavior and body language** – By paying attention to nonverbal cues, nurses can gain a deeper understanding of what patients are trying to communicate.
2. **Repeating back the main point or message** – This helps confirm that the nurse has understood what the patient is saying and gives the patient an opportunity to clarify if there is any confusion.

3. **Clarifying anything that is unclear** – Nurses should ask questions to ensure they fully understand what the patient is saying and avoid misunderstandings.
4. **Reserving judgment** – Nurses should avoid passing judgment on patients and instead try to understand and empathize with their situation.

Verbal Communication

Verbal communication is an essential skill for nurses in order to provide high-quality health services. Nurses must be able to communicate clearly, accurately and honestly with patients and other health care professionals.

To achieve excellent verbal communication, nurses should:

1. **Speak with clarity and accuracy** – This means using proper grammar, pronunciation and enunciation when speaking.
2. **Know their audience** – It is important to understand the person's age, culture and level of health literacy and adjust language accordingly.
3. **Be aware of the tone of voice** – Nurses must be mindful of their emotional state and not let stress or frustration affect patient interactions.
4. **Encourage patients to communicate** – By asking open-ended questions, such as "Can you tell me a bit more about that?" nurses can encourage patients to share their thoughts and feelings.
5. **Avoid condescending pet names** – Instead, use the patient's first name or name of choice.
6. **Speak in clear, complete sentences** – Avoid using technical jargon or medical terms that the patient may not understand.

Nonverbal Communication

Nonverbal communication is just as important as verbal communication in creating a rapport with patients and building trust. Nurses must be aware of the nonverbal cues they are sending and use them to create a positive and empathetic connection with patients.

Some tips for effective nonverbal communication include:

1. **Showing interest** – Maintain eye contact and nod while patients are speaking to indicate that you are engaged and paying attention.
2. **Smiling** – A simple smile can go a long way in creating a positive and welcoming environment for patients.
3. **Avoiding prolonged staring** – While maintaining eye contact is important, staring can be perceived as invasive or uncomfortable.

4. **Sitting down and leaning forward** – When possible, sit down and lean forward when interacting with patients to convey a sense of engagement and attentiveness.
5. **Using nonthreatening body language** – Keep your posture open and avoid crossing your arms or legs, which can convey defensiveness or closed-mindedness.

Written Communication

Effective written communication skills are critical for nurses, as they are responsible for creating and maintaining accurate patient medical records. Other health care professionals use these records to provide the best possible care to patients, so it is essential that they be accurate, current and written in a clear and legible manner.

To improve your written communication skills, you can:

1. **Take notes immediately** – After providing treatment for a patient, make sure to jot down some notes right away so that you do not lose any crucial details.
2. **Write legibly and clearly** – Make sure that your writing is easy to read and comprehend by using clear and direct language.
3. **Note accurate dates and times** – It is essential to include correct dates and times in patient records in order to maintain continuity of care and reduce the likelihood of mistakes.
4. **Protect patient confidentiality** – At all times, maintain strict adherence to patient confidentiality and take steps to safeguard sensitive information.

Conflict Resolution

It is possible for nurses, doctors and other members of the health care staff, as well as patients and health care providers, to find themselves in conflict with one another in a hospital setting.

In order to resolve conflicts effectively in nursing, one must possess a number of critical skills, including:

1. **Active listening** – Nurses can comprehend the viewpoints of all parties involved and discover the underlying issues that are causing the disagreement if they listen intently and actively participate in the conversation.
2. **Empathy** – Nurses can help relieve tension and develop rapport with patients and colleagues if they take the time to empathize with others' experiences and share their own sentiments.

3. **Problem-solving skills** – The ability to recognize and assess problems, think creatively about possible solutions and assess the range of outcomes that could result from those solutions is essential for nurses.
4. **Mediation** – When patients and other members of the health care team have disagreements or conflicts, nurses can step in as impartial third parties to help mediate the situation.
5. **Cultural sensitivity** – It is essential for nurses to be able to recognize and appreciate their patients' and coworkers' various cultural backgrounds.
6. **Communication** – In order to settle problems and maintain strong relationships, RNs need to have the ability to communicate with all parties involved in a way that is both clear and effective.

Information-Sharing

There are several key information-sharing strategies that nurses can use, including:

The **Situation, Background, Assessment and Recommendation (SBAR)** is a tool that assists in providing structure and standardization to the communication that takes place among professionals working in the health care industry. It makes it possible to provide vital patient information in a way that is both clear and succinct.

1. **Situation** – A condensed explanation of the patient's current state and the motivation behind this communication
2. **Background** – Information that is pertinent to the patient's history, such as their diagnosis, any allergies and the medications they are now taking
3. **Assessment** – A description of the patient's current condition, including vital signs, symptoms and any changes in the patient's condition
4. **Recommendation** – A request for action or information that is crystal clear and very explicit, including any necessary follow-up activities or concerns

The SBAR tool may be utilized in a variety of contexts, including patient handoffs, the transfer of care between shifts or units and the solicitation of consultation from other medical professionals. It is made to be straightforward and it helps medical professionals concentrate on the data that is of the utmost significance. As a result, errors are minimized and patient results are enhanced.

SBAR can improve communication while reducing the likelihood of errors. It also helps to ensure that all critical information is shared and that follow-up measures are taken in a timely manner, leading to improved coordination of care. This can be accomplished by ensuring that follow-up actions are taken in a timely manner.

Hand-off – This is the handing off of patient care from one member of the medical staff to another. It is essential that handoffs be carried out in a way that is both transparent and well-organized to guarantee that all pertinent patient information is communicated and that patients continue to receive continuous care.

Closed-loop communication and **check-back** are comparable in that they require following up with the person who supplied the information in order to confirm that it was comprehended appropriately and any necessary follow-up steps have been carried out. Closed-loop communication refers to the overall process of ensuring that information is accurate and complete, whereas check-back refers to following up with the person who provided the information.

In the process of closed-loop communication, in addition to the check-back phase, there are other processes, such as repeating the information that was given, which allows the person who gave the information to verify that it was conveyed accurately. It contains feedback to ensure that the information was acted upon, as well as feedback to the person who provided the information in order to let them know what actions were taken. It also includes feedback to ensure that the information is acted upon.

Read-back – This is a procedure that entails restating the material that was presented in order to verify that it was comprehended in its entirety and that any necessary follow-up steps have been carried out.

Huddle – This is a quick meeting that medical experts hold to discuss pertinent patient information, as well as to plan and coordinate care.

Verbal orders – When a health care worker gives an order verbally rather than in writing, this is called "verbal order taking."

Bedside report – At this point, the nurse will offer a report on the patient's current status, the treatment being administered and any shifts in the patient's overall health.

Interdisciplinary – This refers to the practice of sharing information and working with other medical professionals from a variety of fields to give patients the highest level of treatment that is clinically feasible.

Communication Barriers

There are several barriers to effective communication in the health care setting:

1. **Need for interpreter/translator** – Language problems can make it difficult for patients to communicate effectively with health care professionals. This can lead to misunderstandings, delays in care and ultimately, bad consequences for the patient. The use of interpreters and translators is one technique to help close

this communication gap; however, it is crucial to keep in mind that these individuals are not always present or available.

2. **Physical limitations** – People who have difficulties communicating due to their hearing, vision or speech may find it challenging to do so with health care professionals. This obstacle can be surmounted by using other modes of communication, such as written notes, sign language or assistive technologies.

3. **Cognitive limitations** – Individuals who suffer from cognitive impairments, such as dementia or illnesses related to their mental health, could have trouble comprehending or communicating information. This challenge can be handled by employing strategies, such as using basic language, repetition and visual aids, as well as by incorporating family members or caregivers in the communication process.

4. **Emotional barriers** – Patients and health care workers alike may experience anxiety and have emotional barriers that make it difficult to communicate effectively. This challenge can be overcome by the utilization of active listening, empathy and an approach that does not pass judgment.

5. **Cultural and ethnic barriers** – Patients may come from a variety of cultural or ethnic backgrounds, any of which might make communication and comprehension more difficult. Having knowledge of the patient's culture, employing cultural brokers and gaining a grasp of the patient's views and values are all effective ways to circumvent this challenge.

6. **Background noise** – Background noise can make it difficult to communicate, regardless of whether one is in a bustling hospital or a patient's home. This challenge can be overcome by communicating in a location that is less noisy or utilizing equipment that filters out ambient noise.

7. **Time constraints** – Because health care personnel are frequently pressed for time, there is a possibility that they will not have the time to adequately connect with their patients. This challenge can be surmounted by placing a high priority on communication and ensuring that sufficient time is set aside for it.

De-Escalation Techniques

De-escalation techniques refer to methods used to reduce tension and defuse potentially violent or aggressive situations. These techniques are important for nurses and other health care professionals to know, as they can help keep patients, staff and themselves safe. Some common de-escalation techniques include:

- **Verbal intervention** – This involves using calm and measured language to diffuse a situation. This can include using a calm tone of voice, speaking slowly and avoiding confrontational language.
- **Active listening** – This involves listening actively to patients to understand their perspectives and concerns. This can help build rapport and trust and to identify the underlying causes of a patient's agitation.
- **Empathy** – By showing understanding and sharing patients' feelings, nurses can help defuse tensions and build rapport.
- **Redirecting the patient's attention** – This can involve providing patients with something to distract them, such as a book or a toy or encouraging them to focus on something else.
- **Open-ended questions** – This can be useful in encouraging patients to express their feelings and concerns.
- **Humor** – Humor can be an effective way to diffuse a tense situation, as long as it is appropriate and respectful.
- **Time-out** – This technique involves separating patients from the situation for a short period of time and giving them the opportunity to calm down.
- **Calling for backup** – If the situation is escalating, it is important to call for backup from colleagues or security.

Critical Thinking

Time Management and Prioritization of Care

Time management and prioritization of care involve planning, organizing and prioritizing tasks and responsibilities in order to provide the best possible care for patients.

Prioritizing care – Nurses must be able to identify patients' most critical needs and prioritize care accordingly. This can involve assessing patients' conditions, identifying potential risks and determining the most appropriate interventions.

Time management – Nurses must be able to manage their time effectively in order to ensure they have enough time to complete all of their tasks and responsibilities. This can involve setting deadlines, breaking tasks into smaller components and using time-saving techniques.

Communication and collaboration – Nurses must be able to communicate and collaborate effectively with other health care professionals in order to prioritize care and manage time effectively. This can involve sharing patient information, delegating tasks and working together to develop care plans.

Crisis Situations and Resources

In health care, crisis situations can include medical emergencies, natural disasters and outbreaks of infectious diseases. It is important for health care organizations to have a rapid response team in place to respond quickly and effectively to these crisis situations.

A rapid response team in health care typically includes medical professionals, such as doctors, nurses and paramedics. They are responsible for providing immediate medical assistance and stabilizing patients who are experiencing a medical emergency. They may also provide advanced life support, such as CPR and defibrillation.

Deteriorating patients in health care are individuals who are experiencing a decline in their health status. Early warning systems are used to detect patients who are at risk of deterioration. These systems use various tools and algorithms to identify patients who are at risk of deterioration and alert health care providers.

Examples of early warning systems in health care include:

- The Modified Early Warning Score (MEWS), which uses a combination of vital signs, patient history and lab results to identify patients at risk of deterioration
- The National Early Warning Score (NEWS), which uses similar parameters as MEWS but with a different scoring system
- The Rapid Response Team (RRT), which is activated when a patient's condition deteriorates and requires immediate medical attention

Crisis Management

Crisis management involves being prepared to respond effectively and efficiently to unexpected events or emergencies that occur during surgical procedures. These events can include equipment malfunctions, complications arising from the surgery and even medical emergencies, such as cardiac arrest.

One way for medical-surgical nurses to prepare for crisis management is to stay informed and updated on the latest guidelines and protocols for surgical procedures, as well as to be familiar with the equipment and instruments that are used in the operating room. They should also be trained in emergency medical procedures, such as CPR and basic life support (BLS).

During a crisis, the nurse should be able to clearly and concisely convey information to the surgical team and other health care professionals, such as anesthesiologists and surgeons, and follow their instructions in real time.

In the event of an emergency, the nurse should also be able to take charge and assume a leadership role if necessary. This may include directing other members of the surgical team, communicating with other health care professionals and first responders and making quick and informed decisions to ensure the patients' safety and well-being.

Critical Thinking

Critical thinking is a vital skill that reflects the ability to think independently and make sound decisions based on reasoning and evidence. It includes several key elements, such as self-regulation, problem-solving, analysis, interpretation and inference.

Self-regulation is the ability to monitor one's own thinking and make adjustments as needed. This can include identifying and overcoming biases, considering alternative perspectives and being open to new information and ideas.

Problem-solving is the ability to identify and analyze problems, generate potential solutions and make decisions based on evidence. This can include identifying potential risks, developing care plans and evaluating treatment outcomes.

Analysis involves breaking down information into smaller parts in order to understand it better. This can include reviewing patient data, identifying patterns and trends and interpreting diagnostic test results.

Interpretation is the ability to understand the meaning of information and make connections between different pieces of information. This can include understanding patient symptoms, identifying potential diagnoses and interpreting medical literature.

Inference is the ability to draw conclusions based on evidence and reasoning. This can include making predictions about patient outcomes, identifying potential complications and developing plans to prevent or manage these complications.

Healthy Practice Environment

Workplace Safety

Workplace safety is a critical aspect of health care, as nurses are often exposed to various physical, emotional and environmental hazards on the job. Ensuring a safe work environment is essential for nurses to be able to provide safe and effective care for their patients without undue stress or risk of injury.

Table 26. Workplace Hazards

Aspect of Safety	Description
Physical safety	Protecting nurses from injuries and accidents in the workplace. This includes implementing proper ergonomics, providing PPE and ensuring that equipment and facilities are in good condition.
Emotional safety	Protecting nurses from emotional and psychological stress. This includes providing support for dealing with difficult patients and situations, promoting a positive work environment and addressing issues such as workplace bullying and harassment.
Environmental safety	Protecting nurses from hazards in the physical environment. This includes ensuring proper ventilation and lighting, controlling temperature and humidity and identifying and addressing potential hazards, such as chemical spills or hazardous waste.

Nurse Resiliency and Well-Being

Nurse resiliency and well-being are key aspects of the nursing profession, as nurses often work in demanding and high-stress environments. Studies have shown that nurses who have high levels of resiliency and well-being are better able to cope with the demands of their job and are more likely to have positive outcomes in terms of job satisfaction, mental and physical health and overall well-being.

- One key strategy to improve nurse resiliency is to provide opportunities for self-care and stress management. This may include activities such as exercise, meditation and mindfulness practices. Additionally, nurses should be encouraged to take regular breaks throughout the workday to rest and recharge.
- Another strategy is to foster a supportive work environment. This can be done by providing regular opportunities for nurses to connect with one another and by creating a culture of open communication and collaboration. Managers and leaders can also play a role in promoting a supportive work environment by providing clear guidance and support to nurses and by creating an environment where nurses feel safe to express their concerns and ideas.
- Promoting work-life balance can be done by providing flexible scheduling options and encouraging nurses to take time off when they need it. Additionally, nurses should be provided with resources and support to help them manage their work-life balance effectively.

- Finally, nurses should have access to mental health services, such as counseling and therapy. Nurses are at higher risk for burnout and mental health issues, like depression and anxiety, so it is important to have access to mental health services that are tailored to the unique needs of nurses.

Unintended Consequences

Unintended consequences refer to unforeseen and unintended negative outcomes that may arise as a result of a particular action or decision. Unintended consequences can include a wide range of issues, such as:

- Increased workload and burnout due to staffing shortages
- Reduced patient satisfaction and outcomes due to inadequate staffing levels
- Increased risk of error or injury due to fatigue or overwork
- Negative impacts on nurses' physical and mental health due to stress and high demands
- Reduced job satisfaction and retention rates among nurses
- Impact of new technology on nurses' role and scope of practice

Moral distress, moral injury, compassion fatigue and burnout are all related concepts that can occur as a result of the unique demands and challenges nurses face in their work.

Moral distress refers to the feeling of being unable to act in accordance with one's personal values or moral code, often due to constraints or obstacles in the health care system. This can lead to feelings of powerlessness, frustration and guilt.

Moral injury is a more severe form of moral distress that occurs when an individual experiences a significant moral transgression or betrayal, leading to lasting psychological harm.

Compassion fatigue is a state of physical, emotional and spiritual depletion that can occur as a result of prolonged exposure to the suffering of others. This can lead to a loss of empathy, emotional numbness and a sense of hopelessness.

Burnout is a state of physical and emotional exhaustion, depersonalization and reduced personal accomplishment that can occur as a result of prolonged stress and high demands. This can lead to feelings of detachment, cynicism and a sense of failure.

Resource Allocation

Resource allocation is the process of determining how resources (such as staffing and equipment) will be distributed and used within a health care organization. The allocation of resources can have a significant impact on the quality of care provided to patients and the well-being of health care workers.

Adequate staffing is a critical resource for ensuring safe and high-quality care. Insufficient staffing levels can lead to increased workload, burnout and fatigue among nurses, as well as an increased risk of error and adverse events for patients. It is important for health care organizations to have an appropriate staffing ratio that takes into account the complexity of the patient population and the acuity of their conditions.

Equipment is another important resource in health care. The availability of appropriate equipment and technology can greatly impact the care provided to patients. For example, having the right diagnostic equipment can help in the accurate diagnosis of diseases and injuries, while the availability of advanced medical equipment can facilitate the delivery of complex care. Health care organizations need to ensure they have the necessary equipment and technology to meet patients' needs.

Peer Accountability

Peer accountability refers to the responsibility and accountability that health care workers have to each other in the workplace. It involves holding oneself and one's colleagues accountable for maintaining high standards of care and professionalism, as well as addressing any issues or concerns that may arise.

Peer accountability can take many forms, including:

- Regular performance evaluations and feedback
- Peer review of clinical practice
- Collaboration and consultation with colleagues
- Participation in quality improvement initiatives
- Adherence to professional standards and guidelines
- Reporting of unsafe or unethical behavior

Scope of Practice and Ethics

Scope of Practice and Code of Ethics for Nurses per Local and Regional Nursing Bodies

The scope of practice and code of ethics for nurses are established by professional nursing organizations and regulated by state boards of nursing. They provide guidance on the responsibilities and expectations of nurses in their professional practice, as well as the ethical principles that govern their work.

The ANA Code of Ethics for Nurses is a comprehensive set of guidelines that serves as a framework for nurses to make ethical decisions in their practice. It includes nine provisions that address different aspects of nursing, such as patient care, self-responsibility and professional responsibility, among others. It is considered the foundation of nursing ethics and a guide for nursing practice, education and administration. The provisions include:

- The nurse's responsibility to the patient
- The nurse's responsibility to the profession
- The nurse's responsibility to self
- The nurse's responsibility to others
- The nurse's responsibility to society
- The nurse's responsibility to the environment
- The nurse's responsibility to the health care system
- The nurse's responsibility to other nurses
- The nurse's responsibility to nursing education

The AMSN Scope and Standards of Practice includes a section on Standard V: Ethical Practice. This standard provides guidance on how nurses can adhere to ethical principles in their practice and promote ethical practice within the health care system.

Standard V includes four elements:

1. **Ethical principles and decision-making** – Nurses must be able to identify and analyze ethical issues, use a decision-making process and communicate with other health care professionals about ethical issues.
2. **Ethical considerations in practice** – Nurses must be aware of and adhere to legal and regulatory requirements, professional standards and organizational policies related to ethical practice.
3. **Ethical considerations in patient care** – Nurses must respect patients' rights to autonomy, privacy and confidentiality and must provide care that is respectful, nondiscriminatory and culturally sensitive.
4. **Ethical considerations in nursing practice** – Nurses must promote an ethical work environment, engage in ongoing professional development and contribute to the advancement of the nursing profession.

AMSN Standard V aligns with the ANA Code of Ethics for Nurses and provides additional guidance on how nurses can apply ethical principles in their practice. This standard is intended to promote ethical practice and provide a framework for nurses to use when making ethical decisions in their practice.

Local and regional nursing bodies may also have their own scope of practice and code of ethics for nurses. These documents may reflect the specific regulations and laws in the region and may include additional provisions on issues such as cultural sensitivity, interdisciplinary collaboration and the use of complementary and alternative therapies.

Patients' Rights and Responsibilities

Table 27. Patients' Rights and Responsibilities

Patients' Rights	Patients' Responsibilities
Receive appropriate medical care	Provide accurate and complete information about medical history and current health status.
Have personal and medical information protected	Follow the treatment plan and keep appointments.
Participate in medical treatment decisions	Be respectful and considerate of health care providers and other patients.
Choose health care providers and receive a second opinion	Provide information about any change in health status.
Access medical records	Voice complaints, grievances or compliments about care and treatment or the health care facility or provider.
Know the costs of their care before receiving it	Understand the insurance company's rules and coverage.

Professional Reporting and Resources

Professional reporting and resources for health care providers refer to the guidelines and procedures for reporting ethical issues, the scope of practice violations and unsafe practices in a health care setting.

1. **Ethics** – Health care providers have a professional and moral obligation to report any ethical issues that arise in the course of their work. This may include issues related to informed consent, patient autonomy and confidentiality.

2. **Scope of Practice** – Health care providers are expected to practice within their scope of expertise and any violation of this can be reported. For example, a nurse

who is practicing outside their scope of expertise, such as performing a surgical procedure, should be reported.

3. **Unsafe practice** – Unsafe practice refers to any behavior or action that puts patients or other health care providers at risk. This includes but is not limited to substance abuse, medical errors and lack of infection control.

Policies, Procedures, Regulatory and Licensure Requirements, Standards of Practice and Applicable State, Federal and Local Laws

Policies and procedures for medical-surgical nurses typically cover various aspects of surgical care, such as patient preparation, instrumentation and postoperative care. Some specific examples of policies and procedures for medical-surgical nurses include:

1. **Patient assessment and preparation** – Nurses are responsible for conducting preoperative assessments and preparing patients for surgery. This may include obtaining informed consent, verifying patient identification and ensuring that patients understand the risks and benefits of the procedure.
2. **Instrumentation** – Nurses are responsible for preparing and maintaining the instruments and equipment needed for surgery. This includes ensuring that all instruments are properly sterilized, equipment is in good working order and necessary supplies are readily available.
3. **Intraoperative care** – Nurses are responsible for providing care during the surgical procedure. This may include monitoring the patient's vital signs, administering medications and providing assistance to the surgical team as needed.
4. **Postoperative care** – After the surgical procedure, nurses are responsible for monitoring the patient's recovery, managing postoperative pain and providing follow-up care. They also have to be aware of any complications that might arise and report them to the surgeon and other members of the health care team.
5. **Infection control** – Nurses are responsible for ensuring that infection-control protocols are followed. This may include properly sterilizing instruments, following hand hygiene protocols and maintaining a clean and safe environment in the operating room.
6. **Documentation** – Nurses are responsible for maintaining accurate and up-to-date documentation of the patient's care, including surgical consent, preoperative and postoperative assessment and any complications that may arise.

Regulatory and licensure requirements for medical-surgical nurses vary by state and country but generally include:

- **Education and training** – Nurses must have a nursing degree, such as an associate's degree in nursing (ADN) or a bachelor's degree in nursing (BSN) and have completed an accredited surgical nursing program. In some states, nurses may be required to have a master's degree in nursing (MSN) to work as surgical nurses.
- **Professional certification** – Nurses must pass the National Council Licensure Examination (NCLEX) to become licensed RNs (RN) and may also be required to hold certification from a professional certification body, such as the National Board of Surgical Technology and Surgical Assisting (NBSTSA) or the Certification for Perioperative Nursing (CNOR).
- **Continuing education** – Nurses must meet continuing education requirements to maintain their license and certification. This may include taking continuing education courses or attending professional development conferences.
- **Background check** – Nurses may be required to undergo a background check to ensure they have no prior criminal convictions or other disqualifying information.
- **Professional liability insurance** – Nurses may be required to carry professional liability insurance to cover any potential legal claims that may arise from their practice.

Standards of Practice

The AMSN has developed standards of practice for medical-surgical nurses, which outline the knowledge, skills and abilities that are essential for safe and effective practice in this field.

Table 28. Standards of Practice

Standards of Practice
Assessment
Diagnosis
Outcomes Identification
Planning
Implementation
Evaluation

Professional Practice	
Education	
Leadership	
Research	

Quality Management

Evidence-Based Guidelines for Nursing-Sensitive Indicators

Evidence-based guidelines for nursing-sensitive indicators are a set of recommendations for nursing practice that are supported by research evidence. These guidelines can help nurses provide high-quality care that is tailored to each patient's needs. Some examples of nursing-sensitive indicators that may be addressed by these guidelines include:

- Patient outcomes, such as mortality and morbidity rates
- Patient satisfaction
- Patient safety and quality of care
- Nurse-patient communication
- Nurse staffing levels and workload
- Nurse education and competency
- Nurse burnout and job satisfaction
- Nurse-led care coordination
- Nurse-led interventions to improve patient outcomes

The ANA and the National Quality Forum (NQF) are among the organizations that develop and disseminate evidence-based guidelines for nursing-sensitive indicators. Nurses, nurse practitioners and other health care professionals can use these guidelines to inform their practice and improve patient outcomes.

Quality Standards and Policies

Refer to guidelines and regulations that are put in place to ensure that health care services are provided to patients in a safe and effective manner. These standards and policies are designed to promote quality and safety and to improve the overall patient experience. Some examples of quality standards and policies that may be in place in a health care setting include:

- **Accreditation standards** – Organizations such as The Joint Commission and the Health Care Facilities Accreditation Program (HFAP) set standards for health care organizations to meet in order to be accredited.
- **Clinical practice guidelines** – These guidelines provide recommendations for the diagnosis, treatment and management of specific medical conditions. They are based on the best available evidence and intended to improve the quality of care.
- **Infection-control policies** – These policies are put in place to prevent the spread of infections in health care settings. They may include guidelines for hand hygiene, cleaning and sterilization of equipment.
- **Medication management policies** – These policies are designed to ensure that medications are prescribed, dispensed and administered safely and appropriately.
- **Patient safety policies** – These policies are intended to prevent patient harm and adverse events. They may include guidelines for preventing falls, preventing pressure ulcers and reducing the risk of hospital-acquired infections.
- **Privacy and security policies** – These policies are put in place to protect patients' personal and medical information. They may include guidelines for the handling and storage of patient records, as well as the use of electronic health records.

Continuous Quality and Process Improvement

Continuous quality and process improvement (CQPI) is an approach to health care that focuses on ongoing assessment and improving processes and outcomes. The goal of CQPI is to enhance the quality of care and the overall patient experience and to improve the efficiency and effectiveness of health care delivery.

CQPI projects can take various forms, including gradual or breakthrough improvements, and may focus on a wide range of areas, such as operations, systems, processes, work environment or regulatory compliance. The CQPI process typically includes defining the problem, benchmarking, setting a goal and implementing iterative quality improvement projects.

Common methodologies used in CQPI include:

- Lean: This approach focuses on eliminating waste and maximizing efficiency in health care processes.
- Six Sigma: Six Sigma uses data-driven methods to identify and eliminate sources of variability and error in health care processes.
- Plan-Do-Study-Act cycle: PDSA is a four-step model for testing and implementing change in health care processes.

- Baldrige Criteria: This framework provides a holistic approach to organizational performance and improvement, including health care processes.

Nursing Professional Practice Model

A Nursing Professional Practice Model (NPPM) is a framework that guides the delivery of nursing care and defines the roles, responsibilities and expectations of nurses within an organization. It outlines the scope of practice for nurses and sets standards for professional conduct and behavior.

An NPPM typically includes the following components:

- **Vision and mission statement** – This defines the nursing organization's overall purpose and goals.
- **Philosophy of care** -This outlines the organization's beliefs and values related to nursing practice and patient care.
- **Standards of practice** – These are the expected levels of knowledge, skill and performance for nurses within the organization.
- **Professional development** – This outlines the organization's commitment to ongoing education and professional development for nurses.
- **Research and evidence-based practice** – This component emphasizes the importance of using research and evidence to inform nursing practice and improve patient outcomes.
- **Professional autonomy and accountability** – This component emphasizes the importance of nurses taking ownership of their practice and being accountable for their actions.
- **Interprofessional collaboration** – This component emphasizes the importance of nurses working effectively with other members of the health care team to provide high-quality patient care.

Adverse-Event Reporting

Adverse-event reporting is a process by which health care providers and organizations document, investigate and analyze incidents that result in harm to patients. The goal of adverse-event reporting is to identify and address systems issues that contribute to patient harm and to implement changes to prevent similar incidents from occurring in the future.

Adverse-event reporting typically includes the following steps:

- **Identification** – Incidents that result in harm to patients are identified and reported to the appropriate person or department.

- **Investigation** – An investigation is conducted to determine the root cause of the incident and identify any contributing factors.
- **Analysis** – The information gathered during the investigation is analyzed to identify trends and patterns and to identify opportunities for improvement.
- **Action** – Based on the findings of the investigation and analysis, appropriate actions are taken to prevent similar incidents from occurring in the future. This may include changes to policies, procedures or systems, as well as education and training for staff.
- **Follow-up** – The effectiveness of the actions taken is evaluated through ongoing monitoring and follow-up.

Patient Customer Experience Based on Data Results

Patient customer experience, also known as patient experience, refers to the overall perception and satisfaction of patients with the care and services provided by a health care organization. Data on patient experience can be collected through various methods, such as surveys, interviews, focus groups and observational studies. The data results are used to measure patients' satisfaction, identify areas for improvement and track progress over time.

One way patient experience data is used is through value-based purchasing programs. These programs link a portion of a health care organization's reimbursement to performance on certain quality measures, including patient experience. For example, a hospital may receive a higher reimbursement if their patient experience survey scores are higher than the national average.

The data results of patient experience can be used to inform and improve various aspects of health care delivery, such as:

- Communication and coordination among staff and providers
- Responsiveness of staff to patients' needs and preferences
- Physical environment of care
- Access to care and services
- Care coordination and continuity
- Emotional and psychological support

Service Recovery

Service recovery is the process of addressing and resolving customer complaints and negative experiences to regain customer satisfaction and loyalty. It is a critical component of customer service and customer satisfaction.

Service recovery can take various forms, such as a face-to-face apology, a phone call or a written response. The goal of service recovery is to restore the customer's confidence and trust in the organization and prevent them from leaving for a competitor.

In health care, service recovery can take the form of addressing patient complaints or negative experiences with care or service. It can include a prompt apology, an explanation of what went wrong and steps taken to address the issue and prevent it from happening again.

Project Development

Project development is the process of planning, organizing and implementing a project from start to finish. The project development process typically includes:

1. **Project initiation**: Identifying and defining the project and establishing project goals, objectives and deliverables, along with assembling the project team
2. **Project planning**: Developing a detailed project plan that outlines the tasks and activities required to achieve the project goals and objectives
3. **Project execution**: Implementing the project plan, managing and monitoring progress and addressing any issues or challenges that arise
4. **Project monitoring and control**: Continuously monitoring and controlling the project to ensure it stays on track and on budget
5. **Project closeout**: Completing the project and ensuring that all deliverables have been completed and accepted

Evidence-Based Practice and Research

Legislative and Licensure Requirements

As a nurse in the United States, you are responsible for following important legislative and licensure requirements when conducting evidence-based practice and research. This includes upholding patient privacy and confidential health information as protected by HIPAA, following ethical standards for research as outlined in the Common Rule, adhering to clinical trial regulations set by the FDA and meeting licensure requirements set by the NCSBN.

Additionally, it is crucial to stay committed to ethical research practices, such as obtaining informed consent from patients and minimizing any harm that might come from your research. This means following professional standards set by organizations like the ANA and the Sigma Theta Tau International Honor Society of Nursing.

Evidence-Based Practice Principles

Table 29. EBP Principles

Step	Description
1. Asking clinically relevant questions	Identify a specific and relevant question that needs answering in the clinical setting.
2. Searching for the best available evidence	Find and gather the most recent and relevant research and data to answer the question.
3. Appraising the quality and relevance of evidence	Evaluate the credibility and relevance of the evidence gathered.
4. Integrating evidence with clinical expertise and patient values	Consider the patient's individual needs and preferences and integrate the evidence with clinical expertise to make an informed clinical decision.
5. Evaluating outcomes of clinical decisions	Continuously monitor and assess the effectiveness of the clinical decision and make adjustments as needed.

Research Process

The 10 steps of the quantitative research process are:

1. **Formulating the problem** – Identifying a clear and specific research problem or question to investigate
2. **Reviewing related literature** – Gathering information on existing knowledge and research related to the problem, including relevant theories and previous studies
3. **Developing a theoretical framework** – Creating a framework that guides the research and provides a basis for understanding the relationships between variables
4. **Identifying research variables** – Determining the key variables that will be studied and measured
5. **Formulating research questions or hypotheses** – Defining clear research questions or hypotheses that guide the study and can be tested
6. **Selecting the research design** – Deciding on the appropriate research design for the study, such as a survey, experimental design or observational study

7. **Defining the population and sampling procedures** – Specifying the target population and determining the sample size and methods for selecting participants
8. **Developing a plan for data collection and analysis** – Designing the methods and procedures for collecting and analyzing data, including the use of instruments or tools
9. **Implementing the research plan** – Conducting the research, including data collection and analysis
10. **Communicating findings** – Presenting and reporting the findings and conclusions, including any implications and recommendations for future research

The steps of the qualitative research process are:

1. **Initial literature review** – Conducting a preliminary review of existing literature, focusing on gaining a broad understanding of the topic without over-sensitizing the researcher to key concepts
2. **Refined literature review** – Conducting a more extensive literature review after key concepts emerge, weaving the insights into the analysis
3. **Conceptual development** – Focusing on developing concepts, constructs, models or theories based on the data rather than using a theoretical framework
4. **Emergent variables** – Allowing variables to become evident as data collection proceeds instead of preselecting them for study
5. **Broad research questions** – Starting with broad research questions that become more focused as data are collected
6. **No hypothesis formulation** – Not formulating hypotheses, as is common in qualitative research
7. **Adaptive data collection** – Using guidelines for data collection but being open to changing the direction of the research as dictated by the data

Qualitative research takes a different approach than quantitative research, with a focus on developing concepts and theories based on the data rather than testing preexisting hypotheses. The steps of the qualitative research process allow for a more fluid and adaptive approach to data collection and analysis, which can lead to a deeper understanding of complex phenomena.

Chapter 6: Nursing Teamwork and Collaboration

Delegation and Supervision

Delegation and/or Supervision Practices

In delegation, an RN assigns specific tasks related to patient care to unlicensed assistive personnel while still being accountable for the overall outcome. However, the nurse cannot delegate responsibilities that require nursing judgment, such as the assessment and evaluation of the impact of interventions on patient care. The nurse remains accountable for the patient's overall well-being and must ensure that the delegated tasks are performed correctly and in accordance with established protocols. Delegation is a delicate balance between transferring responsibility and retaining accountability, making it a crucial practice for ensuring high-quality patient care.

Supervision is the process of directing, guiding and influencing the performance of a task. It involves providing guidance or direction, oversight, evaluation and follow-up to ensure the successful completion of a delegated task by assistive personnel. Supervision of patient care is a vital component of the nursing profession and requires the licensed nurse to provide guidance and direction to ensure the best possible outcomes for patients. The individuals engaged in supervision are not considered managerial supervisors under federal labor law.

Table 30. ANA's Principles for Delegation

Principle
1. Nursing profession sets scope and standards.
2. RN holds responsibility and accountability.
3. RN directs care and utilizes resources.
4. RN delegates tasks, not the nursing process.
5. RN considers policies, skills and experience of a delegate.
6. Delegation decision is based on patient care complexity, delegate competence and supervision required.
7. Delegation requires mutual respect.
8. Nurse leaders are responsible for monitoring delegate competence.

9. Organization is accountable for resources and documented competency.

10. Policies are developed with RN participation.

Scope of Practice

The scope of practice for RNs is determined by professional nursing organizations and state/provincial boards of nursing. It outlines the responsibilities, duties and tasks that RNs are qualified and licensed to perform.

Unlicensed team members, such as nursing assistants, may perform tasks delegated by the RN as long as they are within their own scope of practice and competence. These tasks may include:

- Assisting with personal care (e.g., bathing, dressing)
- Taking vital signs
- Repositioning patients
- Collecting specimens for testing

Prioritization Skills

Nurses have a complex and ever-changing work environment, making it vital to have a structured approach to patient care. Effective prioritization skills allow a nurse to allocate their time and resources efficiently to ensure that each patient receives the necessary care. Some key elements of prioritization skills for medical-surgical nurses include:

Assessment – Conducting a thorough assessment of each patient's needs and conditions to determine which patients require the most immediate attention.

Urgency – Identifying the urgency of each patient's needs, such as those with life-threatening conditions and addressing those first.

Multitasking – Being able to manage multiple tasks and patient care needs simultaneously while ensuring that each task is completed efficiently and effectively.

Time management – Allocating the appropriate amount of time to each task and patient while being mindful of competing priorities and the overall workload.

Communication – Collaborating with other health care professionals and effectively communicating with patients and their families to ensure a coordinated approach to care.

Case example -A medical-surgical nurse has just begun his shift and is assigned to care for four patients: Patient A with a recent heart attack, Patient B with uncontrolled diabetes, Patient C with a urinary tract infection and Patient D with a stable chronic condition.

The nurse conducts a thorough assessment of each patient to determine their needs and conditions. He identifies that Patient A is the most urgent case, as she has experienced a heart attack and requires close monitoring. The nurse decides to attend to Patient A first and prioritize her care, ensuring that she is stable and that any necessary interventions, such as monitoring vital signs, administering medication and communicating with the physician, are carried out promptly.

Next, the nurse attends to Patient B, with uncontrolled diabetes, who requires monitoring of blood sugar levels and insulin administration. The nurse also schedules a follow-up with the physician to adjust their medication regimen.

Patient C, with a urinary tract infection, requires prompt treatment, and the nurse administers antibiotics and schedules a follow-up to monitor progress.

Finally, the nurse attends to Patient D, with a stable chronic condition, providing the necessary care, such as monitoring the patient's condition and administering medication, while being mindful of the overall workload.

Budgetary Considerations

Budgeting is a critical aspect of the health care sector and helps establish a clear understanding of revenue and expenditures over a particular period, typically a year. Capital and operating budgets are the two main types of health care budgets that have an impact on nursing practices. Capital budgets are employed to plan and upgrade tangible assets, such as facilities or computers, that change in value over time. Operating budgets, on the other hand, encompass personnel expenses and the yearly operating costs of health care facilities. Approximately 40% of the operating budgets of health care organizations are dedicated to nursing staffing, making it vulnerable to reductions in hours and other cost-saving measures during budgeting constraints.

Health care organizations aim to offer high-quality nursing care at an affordable cost through the use of various staffing strategies, such as utilizing agency nurses during shortages, mandatory overtime, team nursing, on-call and off with benefits, floating and acuity-based staffing.

Supplies – Nurses need access to a variety of medical supplies that can include, but are not limited to, gloves, gowns, masks, needles, syringes, wound dressings and diagnostic equipment. The cost of these supplies must be taken into account when budgeting for nursing care.

Staffing – The cost of staffing is one of the largest expenses for health care facilities. This includes salaries, benefits, training and development programs and agency fees for temporary staffing during shortages.

Fiscal efficiency – Implementing cost-saving measures, such as resource optimization and workflow analysis, can help reduce expenses and improve fiscal efficiency. This can include streamlining processes, reducing waste and finding new, more efficient strategies.

Career Development Relationships

Professional Engagement

Professional engagement for nurses refers to the level of involvement and commitment a nurse has toward professional development and the nursing profession as a whole. This can include continuing education, participation in professional organizations, volunteering and advocacy for patient care and the nursing profession. Engagement in these activities helps nurses stay up to date on the latest developments in their field, connect with other professionals and contribute to the advancement of the nursing profession.

Mentoring and Coaching Resources

Some resources for nurses seeking mentorship and coaching include:

1. **Professional nursing organizations** – Many professional nursing organizations offer mentorship and coaching programs for members.
2. **Hospitals and health care organizations** – Some hospitals and health care organizations have internal mentorship and coaching programs for their staff.
3. **Online communities and forums** – There are online communities and forums where nurses can connect with other professionals and receive mentorship and coaching.
4. **Conferences and workshops** – Conferences and workshops focused on nursing and health care often provide opportunities for nurses to receive mentorship and coaching.
5. **Personal networks** – Nurses can also seek out mentorship and coaching through personal networks, such as colleagues, friends and family members.

Reflective Practice

Reflective practice involves reflecting on experiences in patient care and other aspects of the nursing profession in order to gain a deeper understanding of one's own beliefs, values and actions. This can help nurses identify areas for improvement, enhance their clinical decision-making and provide better patient care.

Reflective practice can be done through a variety of methods, including journaling, debriefing sessions with colleagues, supervision and feedback sessions with a mentor or supervisor and participation in continuing education and professional development programs. The key is to regularly reflect on experiences, consider new information and perspectives and make changes to one's practice as necessary.

Roles and Responsibilities

This topic is covered earlier in the book.

Coaching and Learning Theories

Nurses can use these theories to guide their coaching and learning experiences and to better understand how to effectively support and facilitate the learning and growth of others. Some of the most commonly used theories include:

1. **Adult learning theory** – This theory suggests that adult learners have unique motivations and needs and are more likely to engage in learning when it is directly related to their work and personal goals.
2. **Transformational learning theory** – This theory suggests that individuals can undergo profound and lasting changes in their attitudes, values and beliefs as a result of their experiences.
3. **Cognitive behavioral theory** – This theory suggests that individuals' thoughts, feelings and behaviors are interconnected and that changing one can lead to changes in the others.
4. **Solution-focused theory** – This theory emphasizes the importance of focusing on solutions rather than problems and of working collaboratively with individuals to help them achieve their goals.
5. **Appreciative inquiry** – This theory suggests that individuals and organizations can improve by focusing on their strengths and successes rather than their weaknesses and failures.

Professional Empowerment

Nursing empowerment signifies the ability of nurses to drive and motivate themselves and others toward achieving positive outcomes in their nursing practice and work environment. Empowerment and quality patient care go hand in hand, as an empowered nursing team can positively impact staff morale, increase productivity, reduce staff turnover and associated costs, improve the quality of patient care and enhance patient safety.

To achieve empowerment and deliver quality care, nurses must cultivate their leadership skills, act as catalysts for positive change, continuously upgrade their education and promote the adoption of evidence-based practices. Essential elements that contribute to nursing empowerment include decision-making power, independence, a manageable workload, fairness and appropriate recognition and reward.

Orientation Planning and Preceptor Best Practices

Orientation is an important component of onboarding and professional development, as it helps new nurses quickly learn about their responsibilities, their workplace and the culture of their organization.

Effective orientation planning should include a combination of didactic education, hands-on training and opportunities for new nurses to meet their colleagues and learn about the organization. It should also include opportunities for the new nurse to ask questions and receive feedback on their performance.

Preceptor best practices refer to the principles and techniques that experienced nurses can use to support and mentor new nurses during their orientation and beyond.

Career Development Resources

Career development resources are the various tools, programs and opportunities that nurses can access to help them grow and advance in their careers. Some of the most common career development resources include:

1. **Education and training** – Nurses can take advantage of continuing education and training opportunities, such as workshops, conferences and online courses, to develop new skills and knowledge.
2. **Professional organizations** – Joining professional organizations, such as the ANA or the National League for Nursing (NLN), can provide access to a wealth of career development resources, including networking opportunities, career advancement resources and educational materials.

3. **Mentorship programs** – There are several mentorship programs such as the American Nurses Association Mentorship Program, Academy of Medical-Surgical Nurses (AMSN) Mentorship Program, Hospital-Based Mentorship Programs, Specialty Nursing Associations and Online Mentorship Programs.
4. **Certification programs** – Nurses can pursue certification in specialized areas of nursing, such as oncology, pediatrics or geriatrics, to demonstrate their expertise and enhance their marketability.
5. **Career advancement programs** – Some organizations offer internal career advancement programs, such as leadership development programs or management training, to help nurses grow in their careers and take on new responsibilities.

Professional Development

Professional Nursing Practice and Individual Competencies

Professional nursing practice is the application of nursing knowledge and skills in the delivery of safe and effective patient care. It is a dynamic and evolving field that requires nurses to constantly update their knowledge and skills to keep pace with changes in health care technology, best practices and patient needs.

Individual competencies are the knowledge, skills and abilities that individual nurses must possess in order to provide high-quality care. These competencies are based on established nursing standards and may vary depending on the nurse's area of specialty or practice setting.

Professional Behaviors

Professional behaviors refer to the actions and attitudes that are expected of nurses as they carry out their roles and responsibilities. Those include networking, participating in professional organizations, continuous learning, practicing evidence-based care, collaborating with interprofessional teams, exhibiting ethical behavior and effective communication skills.

Clinical Judgment

Clinical judgment requires nurses to synthesize and analyze information, consider multiple options, weigh potential risks and benefits and make sound decisions that prioritize patient safety and well-being. Key factors that influence clinical judgment include a nurse's level of education and experience, exposure to diverse patient populations and access to current and relevant information.

Peer Review Methods

Peer review is a process in which a nurse's performance and practices are evaluated by other health care professionals. The purpose of peer review is to promote quality improvement, identify areas for improvement and provide feedback to the nurse. Peer review can be a valuable tool for promoting professional growth and development, as well as ensuring patient safety. There are several methods of peer review, including:

1. **Chart audits** – A systematic review of a nurse's documentation to ensure accuracy and completeness.
2. **Direct observation** – A colleague observes the nurse in practice to assess competency and identify areas for improvement.
3. **Case conferences** – A team of health care professionals reviews and discusses specific patient cases to identify best practices and areas for improvement.
4. **360-degree feedback** – A multisource evaluation in which the nurse receives feedback from colleagues, supervisors, patients and other stakeholders.
5. **Incident reporting and analysis** – A systematic review of adverse events to identify root causes and implement changes to prevent future incidents.

Educational Needs Assessment

An educational needs assessment is used to identify areas where nurses may benefit from additional training or education in order to provide safe and effective patient care.

The educational needs assessment process typically includes the following steps:

1. **Identifying the need** – This step involves identifying areas where gaps in knowledge or competencies may exist based on patient care requirements, organizational goals and regulations.
2. **Gathering data** – This step involves collecting data through surveys, focus groups and direct observation of practice.
3. **Analyzing data** – This step involves analyzing the data collected in the previous step to identify areas of strength and areas for improvement.
4. **Developing a plan** – Based on the results of the analysis, a plan is developed to address the identified needs, including the type and duration of education and training required.
5. **Implementing the plan** – The plan is carried out with specific tasks in the documented order to ensure nothing is missed.

Leadership

Regulatory and Compliance Standards

Nurses are regulated and governed by compliance standards and regulations, such as:

1. **The Nursing Practice Act** – This act sets the standards and guidelines for the practice of nursing, including the roles and responsibilities of medical-surgical nurses.
2. **The ANA Code of Ethics** – This code sets ethical and moral standards for nurses, including medical-surgical nurses and guides their professional conduct.
3. **The Joint Commission** – This is a health care accrediting organization that sets standards for patient care and safety and requires medical-surgical nurses to meet specific patient care requirements.
4. **OSHA (Occupational Safety and Health Administration**) – OSHA sets safety standards for health care workers, including medical-surgical nurses, to prevent workplace injuries and illnesses.
5. **HIPAA (Health Insurance Portability and Accountability Act)** – This act sets national standards for protecting the privacy and security of patients' health information, and medical-surgical nurses must comply with HIPAA regulations.

Organizational Structure

The organizational structure can vary depending on the size and type of health care organization but typically includes the following levels:

1. **Staff nurses** – They are responsible for direct patient care.
2. **Charge nurses** – They supervise and coordinate the work of staff nurses and act as a resource to them.
3. **Nurse managers** – They are responsible for overseeing a unit or department and managing the daily operations, including staffing and budgeting.
4. **Director of nursing** – They are responsible for overseeing the entire nursing department, ensuring that patient care standards are met and implementing policies and procedures.
5. **Chief nursing officer (CNO)** – They are the top nursing executives in an organization, responsible for strategic planning and overall management of nursing services.

Shared Decision-Making

Shared decision-making (SDM) is a collaborative approach to health care where patients and their health care providers work together to make treatment and management decisions. The goal of SDM is to involve patients in the decision-making process, taking into account their values, preferences and goals, as well as the best available evidence and clinical guidelines.

The health care provider presents options and the potential risks and benefits of each, while the patient actively participates in the discussion and ultimately decides which option is best for them. This approach is meant to increase patient engagement, satisfaction and adherence to treatment plans.

Nursing Philosophy

A nursing philosophy serves as a framework for guiding nursing practice and decision-making and helps define the scope and standards of nursing as a profession.

A typical nursing philosophy includes beliefs about:

- **The nature of health and illness** – This includes an understanding of health as a holistic state of well-being, taking into account physical, mental, emotional and spiritual aspects.
- **The role of the nurse** – This includes the belief that the nurse's primary role is to provide care and support to patients and their families and to promote health and well-being.
- **The patient-nurse relationship** – This includes the belief that the nurse-patient relationship is built on trust, compassion and mutual respect.
- **The nursing process** – This includes the belief that the nursing process is an iterative and holistic approach to patient care, including assessment, diagnosis, planning, implementation and evaluation.

Leadership Models

Each leadership style has its own strengths and weaknesses and the most effective nurse leaders may use elements of different styles in different situations. Some of the leadership styles are described below.

1. **Transformational** – This leadership style focuses on inspiring and motivating others to achieve a shared vision or goal. Transformational nurse leaders are often seen as visionary and charismatic and they create a positive and supportive work environment.

2. **Servant** – This leadership style focuses on putting the needs and well-being of patients and colleagues first and empowering others to reach their full potential. Servant nurse leaders prioritize the development of their team and they are seen as selfless and compassionate.

3. **Autocratic** – This leadership style focuses on maintaining control and authority and relying on a clear hierarchy of power to make decisions. Autocratic nurse leaders often make decisions quickly and decisively, but they may not take others' opinions into consideration.

4. **Laissez-faire** – This leadership style focuses on delegating responsibility and authority to others and allowing them to make decisions and take action independently. Laissez-faire nurse leaders may provide minimal guidance or support, and they may not be actively involved in the decision-making process.

5. **Shared** – This leadership style focuses on collaboration and teamwork and engaging others in the decision-making process. Shared nurse leaders prioritize inclusive and communicative practices and they build strong relationships with other health care providers and stakeholders.

Nursing Care Delivery Systems

Nursing care delivery systems involve the methods and strategies used to manage and organize nursing care in health care facilities. The most common systems are:

1. **Total patient care (TPC)** – A system in which one nurse is responsible for all aspects of a patient's care

2. **Team nursing** – A system in which a team of nurses works together to provide care for a group of patients

3. **Primary nursing** – A system in which one nurse is assigned to a patient and provides continuous, comprehensive care

4. **Case management** – A system in which a nurse coordinates the care multiple health care professionals provide to a patient

5. **Patient-centered care** – A system in which patients are actively involved in decision-making and goal-setting for their own care

Change Management

ADKAR is a model of change management that provides a framework for understanding and managing change in organizations. The acronym stands for Awareness, Desire, Knowledge, Ability and Reinforcement, and these five elements represent the key steps in the change process:

1. **Awareness** – Understanding the need for change and the potential impact on individuals and the organization

2. **Desire** – Developing a strong desire to support and participate in the change
3. **Knowledge** – Acquiring the knowledge and skills necessary to implement the change
4. **Ability** – Building the ability to implement the change, often through training and coaching
5. **Reinforcement** – Ensuring that the change becomes embedded in the organization through ongoing support and reinforcement

The ADKAR model provides a structured approach to change management, helping organizations ensure that change is implemented effectively and sustainably.

Recruitment and Retention

Recruitment and retention of nurses is a major challenge faced by health care organizations. Recruitment efforts focus on attracting qualified and skilled nurses to fill open positions, while retention efforts aim to reduce turnover and keep experienced nurses on staff. Effective recruitment strategies include offering competitive salaries and benefits, providing opportunities for professional growth and development and creating a positive work environment. To retain nurses, organizations can focus on improving work-life balance, offering support and recognition and addressing burnout and job stress. Additionally, organizations can implement nurse-led initiatives and provide opportunities for nurses to participate in decision-making processes.

Employee Engagement

Employee engagement for nurses implies the level of involvement, commitment and satisfaction that nurses have with their work and workplace. High levels of employee engagement can lead to improved job performance, increased patient satisfaction and reduced turnover. Strategies for promoting employee engagement for nurses may include providing opportunities for professional growth and development, promoting work-life balance, fostering a positive workplace culture and recognizing and rewarding excellent performance.

Staff Advocacy

Staff advocacy is the act of supporting and promoting the rights, interests and welfare of employees in the workplace. This can include advocating for better working conditions, fair compensation and improved access to resources and training. Effective staff advocacy requires strong communication and negotiation skills, as well as a deep understanding of the issues facing employees in the industry. It can involve working with management, union representatives and other stakeholders to address workplace challenges and create positive change for staff.

Conflict Management

This topic is covered earlier in the book.

Financial Stewardship

Financial stewardship is the responsible management of financial resources in a manner that ensures the long-term sustainability of health care organizations while maintaining or improving the quality of care they provide to patients. This involves making decisions and taking actions that balance financial considerations with the needs and well-being of patients, staff and stakeholders.

Examples of financial stewardship in health care include:

1. Budget management
2. Resource allocation
3. Cost control
4. Investment management
5. Performance measurement

Disaster Planning and Management

Emergency Procedures

Emergency procedures refer to the protocols and processes that are followed in the event of a medical emergency. The specific procedures may vary depending on the setting (hospital, clinic, long-term care facility), but they generally include steps to ensure the safety of patients and staff, as well as to provide prompt and effective medical intervention.

Examples of emergency procedures include:

1. **CPR** – A life-saving procedure used to restart a patient's heart and breathing in the event of cardiac arrest
2. **Administration of emergency medications** – Giving medications to treat life-threatening conditions, such as anaphylaxis or cardiac arrest
3. **Activation of emergency response teams** – Notifying the appropriate personnel, such as doctors, paramedics or security personnel, in the event of a medical emergency
4. **Evacuation procedures** – Following established protocols for safely evacuating patients and staff in the event of a disaster or other emergency situation

5. **Documentation** – Recording important information about the emergency, such as patient information, treatments provided and other relevant details

Hospital Incident Command Structure

The hospital incident command structure (ICS) is a system used to manage emergencies and other incidents in a hospital setting. It provides a clear chain of command and a structured approach to coordinating the response of various hospital departments, health care professionals and other stakeholders during an emergency.

The ICS is typically organized into several key components, including:

1. **Command** – A designated individual who is responsible for overall management of the incident and coordination of the response
2. **Operations** – The personnel responsible for carrying out specific tasks and actions to manage the incident
3. **Planning** – The personnel responsible for collecting and analyzing information about the incident and developing strategies for responding to it
4. **Logistics** – The personnel responsible for providing resources and support to the incident response, including supplies, equipment and transportation
5. **Finance and administration** – The personnel responsible for tracking and documenting the expenses related to the incident response, as well as other administrative functions

The ICS is designed to be flexible and adaptable to the specific needs of each incident. It allows for effective coordination of the response effort, ensures that all stakeholders have a clear understanding of their roles and responsibilities and helps minimize confusion and duplicated effort.

Test 1: Questions

(1) What is the role of a trocar in surgical procedures?

(A) It is used to clamp off blood vessels to reduce bleeding

(B) It is a type of retractor used to hold open incisions

(C) It is a device used for suturing incisions

(D) It is a tool used to introduce cannulas or other devices into a body cavity

(2) What is the function of a hemostat in surgical procedures?

(A) To provide a magnified view of the surgical site

(B) To keep incisions open during the procedure

(C) To control bleeding by clamping off blood vessels

(D) To cut through tissue and separate it

(3) A patient on IV antibiotics has been experiencing diarrhea. What could this potentially indicate?

(A) The patient is not absorbing the antibiotic correctly

(B) The patient might be developing antibiotic-associated colitis

(C) The patient is allergic to the antibiotic

(D) The antibiotic is effectively killing bacteria

(4) Which type of diet is designed for patients who have heart failure or kidney disease or are on dialysis?

(A) Clear liquid diet

(B) Full liquid diet

(C) Soft diet

(D) Low-sodium diet

(5) A patient who was recently discharged with an oral antibiotic prescription for a wound infection has called in complaining of mild nausea after taking the antibiotic. What advice should the nurse give?

(A) Stop taking the antibiotic and return to the hospital immediately

(B) Take the antibiotic with a small amount of food, despite instructions to take it on an empty stomach

(C) Continue to take the antibiotic and try to take it with a small amount of food, unless directed otherwise

(D) Discontinue the antibiotic and wait for the symptoms to subside

(6) What is the impact of using high-osmolarity enteral nutrition solutions on the patient's body?

(A) Reduced risk of dehydration

(B) Increased risk of hyperosmolarity

(C) No impact on the patient's body

(D) Improved gastrointestinal function

(7) Which type of enteral nutrition is typically used for patients who have a higher calorie requirement?

(A) Continuous enteral nutrition

(B) Bolus enteral nutrition

(C) IV nutrition

(D) Topical nutrition

(8) What is the typical duration of enteral access through a small-bore nasoenteric tube?

(A) Less than four weeks

(B) More than six weeks

(C) Four to six weeks

(D) None of the above

(9) What is the preferred method of enteral access for a patient requiring long-term nutritional support?

(A) Small-bore nasoenteric tube

(B) Gastroscopy or jejunostomy tube

(C) Continuous enteral nutrition

(D) Bolus enteral nutrition

(10) Which type of enteral access is suitable for short-term use only?

(A) Gastroscopy or jejunostomy tube

(B) Small-bore nasoenteric tube

(C) Continuous enteral nutrition

(D) Bolus enteral nutrition

(11) What is the method used to confirm the placement of an enteral nutrition tube?

(A) Ultrasound

(B) Endoscopic visualization

(C) X-ray

(D) Blood test

(12) What is the main cause of tube obstruction in enteral nutrition?

(A) Overfeeding

(B) Flushing the tube with insufficient water

(C) Insufficient head elevation during feedings

(D) Tube trauma to the insertion site

(13) What is the primary way to prevent aspiration pneumonia in enteral nutrition?

(A) Monitor blood glucose levels.

(B) Monitor electrolyte levels.

(C) Elevate the head of the bed during feedings.

(D) Secure the tube to minimize trauma to the insertion site.

(14) What is the recommended way to monitor for potential GI complications in enteral nutrition?

(A) Check tube placement by X-ray.

(B) Monitor fluid intake and output.

(C) Monitor for diarrhea, delayed gastric emptying and constipation.

(D) Check the pH of gastric secretions.

(15) What is the difference between peripheral venous nutrition (PVN) and central venous nutrition (CVN)?

(A) PVN is delivered through a peripheral vein, such as in the arm or hand, and CVN is delivered through a central vein, such as in the neck or chest.

(B) PVN is typically used for patients who require long-term nutritional support, and CVN is used for patients who require short-term nutritional support.

(C) PVN typically contains higher concentrations of glucose and amino acids compared to CVN.

(D) CVN is a less invasive option compared to PVN and can be administered in a hospital or outpatient setting.

(16) What is the recommended time period for short-term nutritional support through PVN?

(A) More than two weeks

(B) Less than two weeks

(C) More than 10 days

(D) Less than 10 days

(17) A patient with frequent bouts of antibiotic-associated diarrhea asks about taking probiotics. What is the most appropriate response from the nurse?

(A) "Probiotics are unnecessary because they don't have any proven health benefits."

(B) "Probiotics can help restore gut bacteria balance and may reduce the risk of antibiotic-associated diarrhea."

(C) "Probiotics are only used in the treatment of chronic diseases like Crohn's disease."

(D) "Probiotics could worsen your diarrhea, so it's best to avoid them."

(18) A patient who has been prescribed a course of antibiotics is also considering taking a probiotic supplement. When should the patient take the probiotic?

(A) At the same time as the antibiotic

(B) Only after finishing the course of antibiotics

(C) 2-3 hours after taking the antibiotic

(D) Probiotics should be avoided during antibiotic treatment

(19) Can fat emulsions be administered through CVN?

(A) Yes

(B) No

(C) Only in some cases

(D) Only through peripheral veins

(20) What is the typical delivery method for long-term nutritional support?

(A) PVN

(B) CVN

(C) Total nutrient admixtures

(D) Fat emulsions

(21) Which of the following types of catheters is typically used for short-term nutritional support?

(A) Tunneled catheter

(B) Peripherally inserted central catheter (PICC)

(C) Non-tunneled or percutaneous catheter

(D) Implanted vascular access device

(22) Which type of catheter is the least invasive?

(A) Implanted vascular access device

(B) Tunneled catheter (Hickman, Broviac, Groshong)

(C) PICC

(D) Non-tunneled or percutaneous catheter

(23) What is the primary mode of transmission for respiratory infections such as the flu?

(A) Airborne transmission

(B) Contact transmission

(C) Droplet transmission

(D) Vector-borne transmission

(24) Which type of catheter is intended for long-term use and inserted surgically?

(A) Non-tunneled or percutaneous catheter

(B) PICC

(C) Tunneled catheter (Hickman, Broviac, Groshong)

(D) Implanted vascular access device

(25) What is the most invasive type of device for nutritional support?

(A) Non-tunneled or percutaneous catheter

(B) PICC

(C) Tunneled catheter (Hickman, Broviac, Groshong)

(D) Implanted vascular access device

(26) What is the difference between a non-tunneled catheter and a PICC?

(A) A non-tunneled catheter is inserted at the bedside, while a PICC is inserted surgically.

(B) A non-tunneled catheter is intended for long-term use, while a PICC is intended for short-term use.

(C) A non-tunneled catheter is less invasive than a PICC.

(D) A non-tunneled catheter is inserted through a peripheral vein, while a PICC is inserted through a central vein.

(27) What is the most important step for providing individualized nutritional strategies for special populations, such as vegetarians, bariatric surgery patients and elderly patients?

(A) Checking patients' weight and BMI regularly

(B) Educating patients and their families about the appropriate diet, physical activity and lifestyle changes

(C) Referring patients with obesity to a dietitian or a nutritionist

(D) Taking into account the patient's unique nutritional needs

(28) Which of the following should be done for patients with obesity to manage their comorbidities?

(A) Assess the patient's nutritional status upon admission and at least weekly thereafter.

(B) Provide individualized nutritional strategies.

(C) Refer the patient for appropriate management.

(D) Educate the patient and the family about maintaining a healthy diet.

(29) A 45-year-old patient with a history of Crohn's disease has been admitted to the hospital for a flare-up of symptoms. The patient has lost a significant amount of weight and reports decreased appetite and difficulty eating. Which of the following nursing interventions can be implemented to improve the patient's nutritional status and prevent malnutrition?

(A) Assess the patient's weight, BMI, dietary intake and any symptoms of malnutrition or malabsorption.

(B) Provide individualized nutritional strategies, such as a high-calorie, high-protein diet.

(C) Refer the patient to a dietitian or a nutritionist for a more in-depth evaluation and individualized nutrition plan.

(D) Educate the patient and the family about the importance of maintaining a healthy diet and lifestyle.

(30) Mrs. Smith is a 68-year-old patient admitted to the hospital for elective surgery. She has a history of type 2 diabetes, heart disease and obesity, with a BMI of 32. What is an important nursing intervention to consider for Mrs. Smith to improve her nutritional outcomes during her hospital stay and prevent any further comorbidities related to her obesity?

(A) Encourage Mrs. Smith to eat a low-fat diet.

(B) Not worry about Mrs. Smith's nutritional status since she is in the hospital for only a short period of time.

(C) Assess Mrs. Smith's nutritional status upon admission and at least weekly thereafter.

(D) Refer Mrs. Smith to a dietitian only after discharge.

(31) Mr. Salazar, a 65-year-old man with a history of Crohn's disease, will be receiving parenteral nutrition at home due to malabsorption issues. He and his wife, who will be administering the nutrition, are concerned about the potential for complications and want to ensure they understand how to properly care for the equipment and handle the solutions. Which of the following steps should the health care team take to educate Mr. Salazar and his wife on the proper administration of parenteral nutrition at home?

(A) Provide written materials on the equipment and procedures.

(B) Offer a demonstration of the proper handling and storage of the solutions.

(C) Schedule a training session with a specialist in home parenteral nutrition.

(D) All of the above.

(32) A 45-year-old man with a history of stroke was recently hospitalized and started receiving enteral nutrition. He has now been discharged from the hospital and will continue receiving enteral nutrition at home. However, he is having difficulty swallowing the nutrition. What should the health care provider do to help improve the patient's ability to swallow the enteral nutrition?

(A) Provide the patient with a soft diet.

(B) Refer the patient for speech consultation.

(C) Increase the frequency of feeding.

(D) Administer nutrition via the parenteral route.

(33) A 65-year-old patient with a history of stroke is being discharged from the hospital after receiving enteral nutrition through a feeding tube for the past month. The patient's primary care physician wants to ensure the patient's continued good nutrition and health at home. What would be the most appropriate next step for the physician to take?

(A) Refer the patient to a speech therapist for swallowing exercises.

(B) Recommend the patient start self-administering parenteral nutrition.

(C) Provide the patient with a list of local support groups for individuals receiving alternate nutrition.

(D) Refer the patient to a registered dietitian for dietary consultation.

(34) Which of the following medical conditions is not commonly associated with the need for alternate forms of nutrition administration, such as enteral or parenteral nutrition?

(A) Gastrointestinal disorders, such as Crohn's disease or severe short-bowel syndrome

(B) Neurological disorders, such as ALS or brain injury

(C) Infections, such as a cold or the flu

(D) Cancer treatment causing loss of appetite or severe nausea

(35) What is the primary focus of patient-centered care?

(A) The health care provider's needs and preferences

(B) The patient's needs and preferences

(C) The medical treatment plan

(D) The reduction of medical errors

(36) What is the main focus of individualized patient care?

(A) Providing generic care to all patients

(B) Prioritizing the patient's unique needs, values and cultural background

(C) Focusing solely on medical treatment

(D) Prioritizing the health care provider's needs and preferences

(37) What is the recommended duration for hand hygiene using an alcohol-based hand sanitizer?

(A) 5 seconds

(B) 10 seconds

(C) 20 seconds

(D) 30 seconds

(38) Which of the following best describes the appropriate care for a patient with a central line dressing that has become loose and soiled?

(A) Re-secure the dressing with medical tape and clean the area with saline.

(B) Change the dressing immediately using sterile technique.

(C) Leave the dressing as it is until the scheduled dressing change.

(D) Clean the dressing with an antimicrobial wipe.

(39) When flushing a central line, which of the following practices helps prevent infection?

(A) Using a clean technique

(B) Using a 10 ml or larger syringe

(C) Using tap water to flush the line

(D) Flushing the line once a day

(40) Why is the environment significant in effective communication in individualized care?

(A) To create an atmosphere that is conducive to effective communication

(B) To reduce the impact on the patient's comfort level

(C) To increase the patient's focus on communication

(D) To avoid nonverbal cues of discomfort

(41) What is a common mistake made by health care professionals in individualized care?

(A) Using appropriate responses to the patient's comments and questions

(B) Failing to concentrate during the encounter

(C) Not asking patients to clarify their statements if there is something not understood

(D) Exhibiting compassion and empathy toward patients

(42) A 65-year-old patient with advanced-stage cancer is admitted to the hospital with severe pain and difficulty breathing. The patient's daughter, who is a nurse, is the primary caregiver and wants to be involved in all aspects of her father's care. What is the most appropriate action for the medical-surgical nurse to take in regard to the daughter's involvement in the patient's care?

(A) Allow the daughter to make all medical decisions without consulting the health care team.

(B) Provide the daughter with basic information about the patient's condition and instruct her to limit her involvement to emotional support.

(C) Include the daughter in all aspects of the patient's care, including decision-making, but ensure that the health care team is consulted and informed about any changes.

(D) Provide the daughter with education and resources to support the patient's health but limit her involvement in decision-making and treatment planning.

(43) Which of the following best describes what health goals should be in patient-centered care?

(A) Vague and unachievable

(B) Specific, measurable and achievable

(C) Unrelated to the patient's health

(D) Set by the health care provider without the patient's input

(44) A patient has been diagnosed with diabetes and has been advised to control his blood sugar levels. The health care provider has set the following health goal for the patient: "To reduce blood sugar levels to within normal range." Which of the following options best represents an achievable, specific and measurable aspect of this health goal?

(A) To increase physical activity

(B) To reduce stress

(C) To eat a healthy diet

(D) To take medications as prescribed

(45) What is not one of the ANA guidelines for patient-centered care?

(A) Respect for patient autonomy

(B) Compassionate care

(C) Technological advancement

(D) Cultural sensitivity

(46) According to the ANA guidelines for patient-centered care, which of the following best represents the principle of continuity of care?

(A) Providing care that is consistent over time and across different settings

(B) Educating patients and families about their health conditions and treatment options

(C) Working in partnership with patients and their families to develop care plans

(D) Respect patients' right to make decisions about their own care

(47) What is the significance of "Respect for patient autonomy" in ANA guidelines for patient-centered care?

(A) It involves providing care that is consistent over time and across different settings.

(B) It requires being aware of and sensitive to the patient's cultural background.

(C) It emphasizes the importance of respecting the patient's right to make decisions about their own care.

(D) It focuses on educating patients and families about their health conditions and treatment options.

(48) What is the purpose of providing personalized resources to patients?

(A) To help them take an active role in their own care and feel more in control of their health

(B) To provide them with generic information about their health

(C) To evaluate their medical history

(D) To direct them to outside organizations or agencies

(49) How can personalized resources be provided to patients?

(A) By assessing their medical history and individual preferences

(B) By providing brochures and pamphlets

(C) By directing them to outside organizations or agencies

(D) By providing generic information about their health

(50) What is the purpose of measuring patient satisfaction in health care?

(A) To evaluate the performance of individual providers

(B) To determine the financial stability of a health care facility

(C) To identify areas for improvement in the health care system as a whole

(D) To gauge the popularity of a health care facility among patients

(51) Which of the following are the requirements for an advance directive to be considered legally binding?

(A) It must comply with federal guidelines and regulations.

(B) It must be signed by a physician.

(C) It must be created in the event of a terminal illness or injury.

(D) It must comply with state-specific guidelines and regulations.

(52) An elderly patient has recently been admitted to the hospital. She has been experiencing shortness of breath and fatigue, and her condition has worsened over the past few days. The physician explains to her family that she may need to be put on mechanical ventilation to help her breathe. The patient has previously expressed her end-of-life preferences and has a _____ in place.

(A) DNR order

(B) Living will

(C) Health care power of attorney

(D) Physician's directive

(53) Mr. Brown has a document in place that outlines his end-of-life preferences. Which of the following best describes the type of document he has?

(A) Advance directive

(B) Physician's directive

(C) DNR order

(D) Health care power of attorney

(54) Mrs. Lee has recently been admitted to the hospital and is unable to make decisions about her medical treatment due to a stroke. Which of the following documents would be most useful in guiding the health care team in their treatment decisions for Mrs. Lee?

(A) Advance directive

(B) Physician's directive

(C) DNR order

(D) Health care power of attorney

(55) Mr. Patel, who has a DNR tattoo on his chest, was involved in a car accident and was brought to the hospital unconscious. What should the health care providers do in this situation?

(A) Perform CPR.

(B) Refrain from performing CPR and honor the DNR tattoo.

(C) Refrain from performing CPR but seek clarification from Mr. Patel's family or health care proxy.

(D) Perform CPR but seek clarification from Mr. Patel's family or health care proxy.

(56) What is the main consideration when preparing a body for viewing by the family after death?

(A) Adherence to cultural customs

(B) Personal preference of the family

(C) State laws and agency policies

(D) Comfort of the deceased person

(57) In which of the following circumstances should the family be allowed to prepare or assist in preparing the body?

(A) Always

(B) Only in some cultures and circumstances

(C) Never

(D) Only when the death was unexpected or unanticipated

(58) _____ guide the preparation of a body for viewing or release to a funeral home in the event of an unexpected or unanticipated death.

(A) Family preferences

(B) Cultural customs

(C) State laws and agency policies and procedures

(D) Personal beliefs

(59) What is the process when a person decides before death to donate his organs or provide anatomic gifts?

(A) Immediate notification

(B) Pre-death declaration

(C) Advance directive

(D) Family permission

(60) How can an individual indicate her willingness to donate her organs or tissues?

(A) By carrying a donor card or by indicating her preference on her driver's license

(B) By completing a written agreement

(C) By indicating that with a tattoo

(D) By verbal communication

(61) Why is the immediate notification of the physician crucial when organ donation is intended?

(A) To coordinate with the organ-sharing network

(B) To ensure the preservation of the donated organs and tissues

(C) To respect the wishes of the individual and their family

(D) All of the above

(62) A 55-year-old patient has been diagnosed with terminal heart failure and has been admitted to the hospital for comfort care. The patient's health is rapidly deteriorating and the medical team has discussed his end-of-life options with him. Mr. Alessio has expressed that he does not want to undergo any life-sustaining treatments, but he has not yet indicated his wishes regarding organ donation. What is the most appropriate next step for the medical team to take?

(A) Proceed with life-sustaining treatments against Mr. Alessio's wishes.

(B) Notify the organ-sharing network and begin the process of obtaining family permission for organ donation.

(C) Respect Mr. Alessio's wishes and provide comfort care only.

(D) Encourage Mr. Alessio to make a decision regarding organ donation.

(63) A 68-year-old patient named Mrs. Green has been diagnosed with end-stage kidney failure and has been admitted to the hospital for dialysis. The patient has expressed that she does not want to undergo dialysis and has indicated that she would like to be placed in hospice care. Mrs. Green has also indicated that she would like to donate her organs after death. Which of the following steps is most important for the medical team to take next?

(A) Ignore Mrs. Green's wishes and proceed with dialysis treatment.

(B) Notify the organ-sharing network and begin the process of obtaining family permission for organ donation.

(C) Transfer Mrs. Green to hospice care and respect her wishes regarding dialysis.

(D) Encourage Mrs. Green to change her mind about donating her organs.

(64) What is the most important assessment a nurse should make for a patient receiving medication through an epidural catheter?

(A) Monitor the patient's blood pressure every 4 hours

(B) Assess the patient's motor function and sensory level regularly

(C) Check the patient's temperature every 2 hours

(D) Measure the patient's urine output every hour

(65) What is the most appropriate nursing action if a patient complains of a severe headache following removal of an epidural catheter?

(A) Administer a prescribed analgesic and reassess in 30 minutes

(B) Encourage the patient to drink plenty of fluids and rest

(C) Position the patient in a supine position and notify the healthcare provider

(D) Document the headache and continue to monitor the patient

(66) What is a primary advantage of utilizing a multimodal approach to pain management?

(A) It reduces the need for patient monitoring

(B) It allows for lower doses of individual medications, reducing the risk of side effects

(C) It enables the use of only non-pharmacological interventions

(D) It increases the patient's dependence on opioids

(67) A patient with post-operative pain is being managed using a multimodal approach. Which of the following combinations best exemplifies this strategy?

(A) Regular administration of opioids, with additional opioids for breakthrough pain

(B) Administration of acetaminophen, gabapentin, and the use of a patient-controlled analgesia (PCA) pump with morphine

(C) Constant infusion of a single analgesic through a patient-controlled analgesia (PCA) pump

(D) Administration of high-dose opioids, with a non-steroidal anti-inflammatory drug (NSAID) for breakthrough pain

(68) When should a nurse consider repositioning as a non-pharmacological intervention for pain management?

(A) Only if the patient requests to be moved

(B) When pain appears to be related to pressure or poor body alignment

(C) Only when all pharmacological interventions have failed

(D) When the patient reports a pain score of 10/10

(69) A patient reports pain from a sprained ankle. What non-pharmacological intervention could the nurse recommend to the patient?

(A) Applying a heating pad to the ankle

(B) Wrapping the ankle tightly with an elastic bandage

(C) Applying a cold pack to the ankle

(D) Performing range of motion exercises with the ankle

(70) A patient asks the nurse about acupuncture as a pain management technique. What should the nurse accurately convey about acupuncture?

(A) Acupuncture is a scientifically unsupported and potentially dangerous treatment method

(B) Acupuncture is a treatment that can only be used for musculoskeletal pain

(C) Acupuncture can be a beneficial complement to traditional pain management strategies for some patients

(D) Acupuncture has no side effects and can replace pharmacological interventions for pain management

(71) What is an important consideration a nurse should advise a patient who wants to try acupuncture for pain management?

(A) Ensure the acupuncturist is licensed and follows safe, clean needle practices

(B) Try self-acupuncture at home before seeing a professional

(C) Stop all other pain management interventions when starting acupuncture

(D) Understand that acupuncture will provide immediate and long-lasting relief from all types of pain

(72) A patient asks about the use of aromatherapy for anxiety relief. What should the nurse keep in mind when responding to the patient's query?

(A) Aromatherapy is an evidence-based therapy for the treatment of serious psychiatric conditions.

(B) There is no evidence that aromatherapy provides any benefits for patients.

(C) Aromatherapy may provide subjective relief of mild symptoms of anxiety for some individuals.

(D) Aromatherapy is generally used as the sole treatment for all forms of anxiety.

(73) When considering the use of aromatherapy for a patient, what is an important safety consideration the nurse should bear in mind?

(A) All essential oils are safe for direct skin contact.

(B) Essential oils can be ingested for faster symptom relief.

(C) Some patients may have allergic reactions to certain essential oils.

(D) There is no risk of interaction between essential oils and pharmaceutical drugs.

(74) Which of the following are required in order to bury or cremate the deceased?

(A) Death certificates

(B) Legal and ethical considerations

(C) Death registers

(D) Burial or cremation permits

(75) When must a death certificate be obtained for a deceased individual?

(A) As soon as possible

(B) After the death is reported to the authorities

(C) After the burial or cremation permit is obtained

(D) After the death is registered with the local government

(76) What is the primary purpose of obtaining a death certificate?

(A) To notify the next of kin

(B) To report the death to the appropriate authorities

(C) To provide official documentation of the cause, time and the deceased's personal details

(D) To obtain a burial or cremation permit

(77) Which medication has been shown to contribute to malnutrition by decreasing appetite and lessening nutrient absorption?

(A) Aspirin

(B) Cisplatin

(C) Amoxicillin

(D) Warfarin

(78) Which type of diet is designed for patients who need a low-residue diet before or after a medical procedure?

(A) Clear liquid diet

(B) Full liquid diet

(C) Soft diet

(D) Low-residue diet

(79) What is the main objective of formulating and writing outcome/goal statements in patient care?

(A) To determine appropriate nursing interventions

(B) To implement the care plan

(C) To evaluate the outcomes and nursing care

(D) To identify the patient's goals and expected outcomes, as well as steps to achieve them

(80) What is the main responsibility of a nurse during the implementation phase of patient care?

(A) To evaluate the outcomes and nursing care

(B) To formulate and write outcome/goal statements

(C) To deliver care to the patient

(D) To gather data about the patient

(81) What is the main objective of evaluating the outcomes and nursing care in patient care?

(A) To determine if the patient's goals have been met

(B) To gather data about the patient

(C) To implement the care plan

(D) To formulate and write outcome/goal statements

(82) What is the nurse's main focus during the assessment phase of the nursing process?

(A) To gather as much information as possible about the patient's health status and needs

(B) To form nursing interventions based on the patient's condition

(C) To evaluate the patient's progress

(D) To perform a physical assessment only

(83) A patient with a portacath complains of pain during a saline flush. What should be the nurse's immediate response?

(A) Administer a painkiller and continue the flush

(B) Stop the flush and assess the patient and the device

(C) Encourage the patient to relax and continue the flush

(D) Increase the speed of the flush to finish it quickly

(84) A patient with a portacath requires a CT scan with IV contrast. What is an important consideration for the nurse preparing this patient for the procedure?

(A) The portacath cannot be used for the administration of contrast media

(B) The portacath needs to be accessed using a non-coring (Huber) needle

(C) The portacath should be removed prior to the procedure

(D) The patient should be given prophylactic antibiotics prior to the procedure

(85) A patient has been admitted to the hospital for chest pain. What is the nurse's first step in the assessment process?

(A) Administering pain medication

(B) Completing a thorough health and medical history

(C) Performing a physical assessment

(D) Noting diagnostic test results

(86) Which type of information is considered subjective information during the nursing assessment process?

(A) Vital signs and diagnostic test results

(B) The patient's health and medical history

(C) The nurse's observation of the patient's physical appearance

(D) All of the above

(87) What is clinical reasoning?

(A) A method of organizing assessment findings

(B) The process of making an appropriate diagnosis

(C) The process of taking vital signs

(D) The process of administering medication

(88) What is the purpose of the PES system in clinical reasoning?

(A) To administer medication to patients

(B) To take patients' vital signs

(C) To organize and communicate assessment findings

(D) To determine the underlying cause of a problem

(89) What is the first element of the PES system in clinical reasoning?

(A) Etiology

(B) Symptoms

(C) Problem

(D) Pathology

(90) The etiology element of the PES system in clinical reasoning represents _____,

(A) The symptoms that the nurse observed during the assessment

(B) The underlying cause or contributor to the problem

(C) A brief nursing diagnosis label

(D) The defining characteristics phrase

(91) What are the steps in identifying patterns and symptoms in nursing assessments?

(A) Ask questions, validate information and analyze symptoms.

(B) Highlight important symptoms, create a list of symptoms and cluster together similar symptoms.

(C) Analyze and interpret symptoms and select a suitable nursing diagnosis label from the NANDA-I list.

(D) All of the above.

(92) A patient has been admitted to the hospital with symptoms of chest pain and shortness of breath. The nurse has completed a thorough health and medical history and performed a physical assessment. What should the nurse do next in the assessment process according to the steps of identifying patterns and symptoms?

(A) Administer pain medication.

(B) Cluster together the symptoms of chest pain and shortness of breath.

(C) Analyze and interpret the symptoms of chest pain and shortness of breath.

(D) Select a suitable nursing diagnosis label from the NANDA-I list.

(93) What is the purpose of using the ABC approach in prioritizing nursing diagnoses?

(A) To address non-life-threatening needs first

(B) To prioritize needs based on the patient's current symptoms

(C) To address life-threatening needs first

(D) To prioritize needs based on the nurse's personal preference

(94) How can a nurse prioritize nursing diagnoses according to Maslow's hierarchy of needs?

(A) By addressing the patient's spiritual needs first

(B) By addressing the patient's physiological needs first

(C) By addressing the patient's self-actualization needs first

(D) By addressing the patient's esteem needs first

(95) In the planning phase of the nursing process, what are the two key factors that should be considered when determining appropriate patient-specific outcomes and interventions?

(A) Patient history and demographics

(B) ABC approach and Maslow's hierarchy of needs

(C) Nurse experience and expertise

(D) Availability of resources and equipment

(96) What is the main focus of the implementation phase of the nursing process?

(A) Curing the underlying medical condition

(B) Managing symptoms

(C) Providing emotional support

(D) Assisting the patient with activities of daily living

(97) What is the role of the nurse during the implementation phase of the nursing process?

(A) Writing the care plan

(B) Monitoring the patient's progress

(C) Carrying out individualized interventions

(D) All of the above

(98) What is the purpose of proper documentation in the evaluation phase?

(A) To provide quality care

(B) To protect the facility and nurse in case of legal dispute

(C) To serve as a legal requirement

(D) To benefit the entire health care team

(99) What is the purpose of problem-oriented charting?

(A) To evaluate care and patient outcomes as part of charting

(B) To serve as a legal requirement

(C) To protect the facility and nurse in case of legal dispute

(D) To benefit the entire health care team

(100) What is the main purpose of evaluation in the nursing process?

(A) To provide quality care

(B) To protect the facility and nurse in case of legal dispute

(C) To reassess patients and compare their condition before and after interventions

(D) To document nursing activities and outcomes

(101) What is the purpose of reviewing documentation with staff during coaching?

(A) To provide feedback and identify areas for improvement

(B) To understand the importance of documentation in patient care

(C) To comply with regulatory requirements related to documentation

(D) To improve the quality and completeness of documentation

(102) What is the importance of training health care professionals on the proper use of technology and equipment?

(A) To familiarize them with the features and capabilities of the technology and equipment

(B) To document patient care in a clear, concise and accurate manner

(C) To improve the quality and completeness of documentation

(D) To minimize the impact of system outages on patient care

(103) Which of the following should health care professionals be familiar with when it comes to technology and equipment use?

(A) How to document patient care in a clear, concise and accurate manner

(B) The features and capabilities of the technology and equipment

(C) How to navigate the system and enter data

(D) All of the above

(104) Which of the following is an example of a healthcare-associated infection (HAI)?

(A) Urinary tract infection (UTI) acquired in the community

(B) Surgical site infection (SSI) after an elective surgery

(C) Influenza contracted from a family member

(D) Food poisoning from contaminated food

(105) What should health care professionals be familiar with when it comes to troubleshooting technology and equipment problems?

(A) The contact information for technical support

(B) The troubleshooting procedures for the technology and equipment

(C) How to reach out for technical support

(D) All of the above

(106) What is the benefit of knowing how to reach out for technical support when troubleshooting technology and equipment problems?

(A) Complying with regulatory requirements related to documentation

(B) Providing the best possible care to patients

(C) Quickly and effectively resolving problems

(D) Learning new troubleshooting procedures

(107) What are EHRs?

(A) Medical records stored on paper

(B) Records that are becoming increasingly popular in providing real-time access to patient information

(C) A type of telehealth service

(D) Documents not used in health care

(108) What is the purpose of telehealth?

(A) To provide in-person health care services

(B) To provide remote health care services, such as telemedicine, teleconsultation and remote patient monitoring

(C) It is not used in health care

(D) To provide medical devices to patients

(109) What is the role of artificial intelligence (AI) in health care?

(A) AI is not used in health care.

(B) AI is used to improve the accuracy and speed of diagnoses, support decision-making and automate routine tasks.

(C) AI is used to monitor patients' vital signs.

(D) AI is used to perform surgeries in health care.

(110) What is IoT, and how is it used in health care?

(A) IoT is a technology that connects various devices, allowing for the collection and analysis of real-time data.

(B) IoT is used in health care to connect medical devices and enable the collection and analysis of real-time patient data, allowing health care providers to make more informed decisions.

(C) IoT is a software system used in health care to manage patient appointments and billing.

(D) IoT is not used in the health care industry.

(111) What is the purpose of robotics in health care?

(A) To perform surgeries and assist in patient care, including rehabilitation and physical therapy

(B) To manage patient appointments and billing

(C) Not used in the health care industry

(D) To provide remote health care services

(112) What is nursing informatics?

(A) The combination of nursing science, computer science and information science that focuses on the use of technology and information to improve patient care

(B) A system for tracking patient data and care plans

(C) A technology used for collecting and analyzing patient data

(D) A platform for conducting research on patient care

(113) What is one of the responsibilities of nursing informatics professionals?

(A) Conducting research on the use of technology and information systems in patient care

(B) Ensuring the use of technology and information systems in patient care complies with relevant standards and regulations

(C) Providing direct patient care

(D) Administering medications

(114) What is the main responsibility of a charge nurse in the nursing chain of command?

(A) Providing direct patient care

(B) Supervising staff and managing specific units or departments

(C) Conducting research on patient care

(D) Ensuring compliance with standards and regulations

(115) What is the chain of command in nursing?

(A) A set of rules and regulations governing the nursing profession

(B) A hierarchy of leadership and authority within the nursing profession

(C) A system of reporting and decision-making within the nursing profession

(D) None of the above

(116) Who is responsible for providing direct patient care in the chain of command of nursing?

(A) The chief nursing officer (CNO)

(B) Nursing managers and directors

(C) Charge nurses

(D) Nurse technicians and staff nurses

(117) What is the main purpose of the chain of command in nursing?

(A) To provide direct patient care

(B) To ensure that decisions are made at the appropriate level

(C) To supervise staff

(D) To manage specific units or departments

(118) What is the primary role of entry-level positions in the nursing chain of command?

(A) Supervising staff and managing specific units or departments

(B) Providing direct patient care

(C) Analyzing data and making evidence-based decisions

(D) Overall nursing strategy and decision-making

(119) What is active listening in nursing?

(A) A technique for avoiding misunderstandings

(B) A method of observing a patient's behavior

(C) A communication skill that involves paying attention and understanding the message

(D) A technique for reserving judgment

(120) What is the benefit of using active listening techniques in nursing?

(A) Improved patient outcomes

(B) Opportunity for the nurse to clarify confusion

(C) A deeper understanding of the patient's needs and experiences

(D) All of the above

(121) What is an active listening technique that nurses can use?

(A) Observing the speaker's behavior and body language

(B) Repeating back the main point or message

(C) Clarifying anything that is unclear

(D) All of the above

(122) What is the importance of verbal communication in nursing?

(A) To confuse patients and health care professionals

(B) To provide high-quality health service

(C) To use technical jargon

(D) To discourage patients from communicating

(123) Which of the following should nurses consider when speaking to patients?

(A) Speaking with clarity and accuracy

(B) Knowing the audience

(C) Being aware of their tone of voice

(D) All of the above

(124) What is one way that nurses can encourage patients to communicate?

(A) Using pet names

(B) Speaking in technical jargon

(C) Asking open-ended questions

(D) Speaking fast

(125) What is the importance of nonverbal communication in nursing?

(A) To ignore patients

(B) To create a rapport with patients and build trust

(C) To transfer patients

(D) To make patients uncomfortable

(126) What is an effective way to show interest in nonverbal communication?

(A) Avoid eye contact

(B) Stare at patients

(C) Maintain eye contact and nod your head

(D) Use threatening body language

(127) What is an example of nonthreatening body language in nonverbal communication?

(A) Crossing arms or legs

(B) Staring at patients

(C) Using an open posture

(D) Ignoring patients

(128) What is the primary purpose of written communication skills for nurses?

(A) To provide entertainment to patients

(B) To record accurate and legible patient medical records

(C) To maintain patient confidentiality

(D) To provide detailed descriptions of patient care

(129) Which of the following should nurses do to improve their written communication skills?

(A) Write in complex language.

(B) Wait until the end of the day to take notes.

(C) Include inaccurate dates and times in patient records.

(D) Take notes immediately and write legibly and clearly.

(130) What is the most important aspect of patient medical records for nurses to maintain?

(A) Legibility of writing

(B) Use of simple language

(C) Accuracy of information

(D) Protection of patient confidentiality

(131) What is the first step in effective conflict resolution in nursing?

(A) Mediation

(B) Cultural sensitivity

(C) Active listening

(D) Empathy

(132) Which roles can nurses play in resolving conflicts in a health care setting?

(A) Neutral third parties

(B) Managers

(C) Transferers

(D) Advocates

(133) A nurse is faced with a conflict between a patient and a physician. Which of the following skills should the nurse first use to resolve the conflict?

(A) Cultural sensitivity

(B) Communication

(C) Active listening

(D) Problem-solving skills

(134) A patient is upset with the care he received from a nurse. Which of the following skills should the nurse use to resolve the conflict with the patient?

(A) Empathy

(B) Cultural sensitivity

(C) Active listening

(D) All of the above

(135) What is the purpose of the SBAR tool in health care communication?

(A) To reduce the risk of errors

(B) To improve the coordination of care

(C) To focus on the most important information

(D) All of the above

(136) Which of the following types of information is included in the Assessment section of the SBAR tool?

(A) Relevant information about the patient's history

(B) A clear and specific request for action

(C) A description of the patient's current condition

(D) A brief statement of the patient's condition

(137) What is the purpose of hand-off in the health care setting?

(A) To transfer patient care from one health care professional to another

(B) To conduct a brief meeting to share important patient information

(C) To ensure that all relevant patient information is passed on

(D) To give the order verbally rather than in writing

(138) What is the main difference between closed-loop communication and check-back?

(A) Closed-loop communication involves repeating the information provided, while check-back specifically refers to the act of following up with the person who provided the information.

(B) Check-back involves repeating the information provided, while closed-loop communication specifically refers to the act of following up with the person who provided the information.

(C) Closed-loop communication and check-back refer to the same process.

(D) Check-back involves repeating the information provided, while closed-loop communication is a process that involves giving feedback to the person who provided the information.

(139) What is a common de-escalation technique that health care professionals use to reduce tension in potentially violent or aggressive situations?

(A) Yelling back

(B) Ignoring the patient

(C) Verbal intervention

(D) Physical force

(140) What is the main objective of time management and prioritization of care in nursing?

(A) To complete all tasks and responsibilities in the shortest amount of time

(B) To prioritize care based on patients' conditions and potential risks

(C) To manage time by creating schedules and delegating tasks

(D) To communicate and collaborate effectively with other health care professionals

(141) What is an example of an early warning system used to detect patients at risk of deterioration?

(A) The Modified Early Warning Score

(B) The National Early Warning Score

(C) The Rapid Response Team

(D) All of the above

(142) What are the key elements of critical thinking in health care?

(A) Self-regulation and interpretation

(B) Problem-solving and inference

(C) Analysis and problem-solving

(D) Self-regulation, problem-solving, analysis, interpretation and inference

(143) Workplace safety in health care is concerned with _____.

(A) Physical safety

(B) Emotional safety

(C) Environmental safety

(D) All of the above

(144) What is the main strategy to improve nurse resiliency and well-being in the nursing profession?

(A) Encouraging nurses to take regular breaks throughout the workday

(B) Providing opportunities for self-care and stress management, such as exercise and meditation

(C) Fostering a supportive work environment through open communication and collaboration

(D) Providing mental health services, such as counseling and therapy

(145) What is the main characteristic of burnout?

(A) Physical and emotional exhaustion

(B) Increased personal accomplishment

(C) Emotional numbness

(D) Sense of hope

(146) What is the main focus of resource allocation in health care organizations?

(A) The allocation of equipment

(B) The allocation of staffing

(C) The allocation of technology

(D) The allocation of patient care

(147) Which of the following elements is included in Standard V of nursing ethics?

(A) Ethical principles and decision-making

(B) Ethical considerations in practice

(C) Ethical considerations in patient care

(D) All of the above

(148) What is the responsibility of a patient in terms of health care?

(A) Receive appropriate medical care

(B) Provide accurate and complete information about medical history and current health status

(C) Follow the treatment plan and keep appointments

(D) Voice complaints, grievances or compliments about care and treatment

(149) What do the AMSN's standards of practice for medical-surgical nurses encompass?

(A) Assessment, diagnosis and outcomes identification

(B) Planning, implementation and evaluation

(C) Professional practice, education and leadership

(D) All of the above

(150) What is the fifth step in the quantitative research process?

(A) Formulating the problem

(B) Reviewing related literature

(C) Formulating research questions or hypotheses

(D) Selecting the research design

Test 1: Answers & Explanations

(1) (D) It is a tool used to introduce cannulas or other devices into a body cavity

A trocar is a surgical instrument that includes a sharp-pointed metal pin enclosed in a tube. It is used to puncture the wall of a body cavity to introduce cannulas or other devices, often during laparoscopic procedures.

(2) (C) To control bleeding by clamping off blood vessels

A hemostat, also known as a hemostatic clamp, is a surgical tool used during surgery to control bleeding. They work by clamping off blood vessels, thus preventing or minimizing blood loss during surgical procedures. While they are often used to clamp blood vessels, they can also be used to grasp and hold tissue.

(3) (B) The patient might be developing antibiotic-associated colitis

While diarrhea can be a common side effect of antibiotic use, severe or persistent diarrhea could be a sign of antibiotic-associated colitis, caused by an overgrowth of the bacteria Clostridioides difficile. This can be a serious condition requiring medical intervention. Other symptoms may include abdominal cramping and fever.

(4) (D) Low-sodium diet.

The goal of this type of diet is to decrease the amount of sodium in the patient's diet to decrease the risk of fluid retention and hypertension. Excess sodium intake can cause fluid buildup, which can be harmful to individuals with heart or kidney problems.

(5) (C) Continue to take the antibiotic and try to take it with a small amount of food, unless directed otherwise

While certain antibiotics should be taken on an empty stomach for optimal absorption, mild nausea is a common side effect of many antibiotics, and taking them with a small amount of food can help alleviate this. However, if the instructions specifically say to take on an empty stomach, the patient should consult with their healthcare provider for personalized advice. Discontinuing an antibiotic prematurely can lead to antibiotic resistance and failure to treat the infection effectively. Severe or persistent symptoms, however, should be reported to the healthcare provider.

(6) (B) Increased risk of hyperosmolarity.

High-osmolarity enteral nutrition solutions have a high concentration of dissolved substances and can have a negative impact on the patient's body by increasing the risk of hyperosmolarity. This condition occurs when the concentration of solutes in the gut is too high, leading to a fluid shift from the bloodstream into the gut, leading to dehydration and other serious complications.

(7) (B) Bolus enteral nutrition.

Bolus enteral nutrition is typically used for patients who have a higher calorie requirement or who are unable to tolerate continuous enteral nutrition. This type of enteral nutrition delivers a larger volume of nutrition in smaller, more frequent doses, helping meet the patient's nutritional needs.

(8) (A) Less than four weeks.

Small-bore nasoenteric tubes are suitable for short-term enteral access, lasting for less than four weeks. These tubes are typically used when enteral nutrition is needed for a brief period of time.

(9) (B) Gastroscopy or jejunostomy tube.

Gastroscopy or jejunostomy tubes are required for long-term enteral access, lasting for more than six weeks. These tubes are preferred for patients who need enteral nutrition for an extended period of time, as they provide reliable and durable access to the gastrointestinal tract.

(10) (B) Small-bore nasoenteric tube.

Small-bore nasoenteric tubes are suitable for short-term enteral access, lasting for less than four weeks. These tubes are typically used when enteral nutrition is needed for a brief period of time and are not recommended for long-term use.

(11) (C) X-ray.

The placement of the enteral nutrition tube is confirmed by X-ray or direct visualization if inserted endoscopically. Ultrasounds and blood tests are not commonly used for confirming the placement of an enteral nutrition tube.

(12) (B) Flushing the tube with insufficient water.

Tube obstruction in enteral nutrition is the main cause of tube obstruction in enteral nutrition. To prevent this, it is recommended to gently flush the tube with 30 mL of warm water before and after feedings.

(13) (C) Elevate the head of the bed during feedings.

The primary way to prevent aspiration pneumonia in enteral nutrition is to elevate the head of the bed 30 degrees during feedings. This helps prevent the flow of enteral nutrition into the lungs, reducing the risk of pneumonia.

(14) (C) Monitor for diarrhea, delayed gastric emptying and constipation.

The recommended way to monitor for potential GI complications in enteral nutrition is to monitor for diarrhea, delayed gastric emptying and constipation. These symptoms may indicate that there are issues with enteral nutrition and prompt further investigation or adjustment of the nutrition plan.

(15) (A) PVN is delivered through a peripheral vein, such as in the arm or hand, and CVN is delivered through a central vein, such as in the neck or chest.

PVN is delivered through a peripheral vein and is typically used for patients who require short-term nutritional support for a period of up to two weeks. CVN is delivered through a central vein, such as in the neck or chest, and is typically used for patients who require long-term nutritional support, as it allows for more consistent and controlled delivery of nutrients.

(16) (B) Less than two weeks.

This method is typically used for patients who require short-term nutritional support for a period of up to two weeks.

(17) (B) "Probiotics can help restore gut bacteria balance and may reduce the risk of antibiotic-associated diarrhea."

Probiotics are live bacteria and yeasts that are good for health, especially the digestive system. While more research is needed to determine the extent of their health benefits, some studies have suggested that probiotics may help prevent antibiotic-associated diarrhea by restoring the balance of gut bacteria disrupted by antibiotic treatment.

(18) (C) 2-3 hours after taking the antibiotic

While probiotics can be beneficial during antibiotic treatment, they should not be taken at the exact same time, as the antibiotic could kill the probiotic organisms. A common recommendation is to take the probiotics at least 2-3 hours after the antibiotic, to allow the antibiotic to be absorbed and lessen its impact on the probiotic organisms. As always, it is important to discuss any supplements, including probiotics, with a healthcare provider to ensure they are safe and appropriate for the individual's specific situation.

(19) (A) Yes.

Fat emulsions can provide essential fatty acids and be administered through either peripheral or central veins.

(20) (B) CVN.

This method is typically used for patients who require long-term nutritional support, as it allows for more consistent and controlled delivery of nutrients.

(21) (C) Non-tunneled or percutaneous catheter.

It is inserted at the bedside and is typically used for short-term nutritional support for up to a few weeks.

(22) (D) Non-tunneled or percutaneous catheter.

This is the less invasive option compared to the other catheter types.

(23) (C) Droplet transmission

Respiratory infections such as the flu are primarily transmitted through droplets generated when an infected person coughs, sneezes, or talks. These droplets can travel short distances and are the main mode of transmission for respiratory infections.

(24) (C) Tunneled catheter (Hickman, Broviac, Groshong).

This type of catheter is intended for long-term use and is inserted surgically.

(25) (D) Implanted vascular access device.

This type of device is surgically implanted and contains no external parts, making it the most invasive but also the most secure and long-term option for nutritional support.

(26) (C) A non-tunneled catheter is less invasive than a PICC.

A non-tunneled catheter is inserted at the bedside and is typically used for short-term nutritional support, while a PICC is inserted through a peripheral vein and is intended for short-term use. A PICC is more invasive than a non-tunneled catheter.

(27) (D) Taking into account the patient's unique nutritional needs.

Special populations, such as vegetarians, bariatric surgery patients and elderly patients, have unique nutritional needs and require special attention to ensure they are getting the nutrients they need. Individualized nutritional strategies should take these unique needs into account.

(28) (C) Refer the patient for appropriate management.

Monitoring patients with obesity for the development of comorbidities, such as diabetes, hypertension and cardiovascular disease and referring them for appropriate management is an important step in managing their health.

(29) (C) Refer the patient to a dietitian or a nutritionist for a more in-depth evaluation and individualized nutrition plan.

This patient is at high risk for malnutrition due to the disease's impact on nutrient absorption. A referral to a dietitian or nutritionist will allow for a comprehensive evaluation of the patient's nutritional status and the development of a personalized nutrition plan to address any deficiencies and prevent malnutrition.

(30) (C) Assess Mrs. Smith's nutritional status upon admission and at least weekly thereafter.

As a patient with obesity and a history of related comorbidities, it is crucial to monitor Mrs. Smith's nutritional status during her hospital stay to ensure that she is getting the nutrients she needs and prevent any further health problems.

(31) (D) All of the above.

The health care team should take a comprehensive approach to educate the patient and his wife on the proper administration of parenteral nutrition at home. This includes providing written materials on the equipment and procedures, offering a demonstration on the proper handling and storage of the solutions and scheduling a training session with a specialist in home parenteral nutrition.

(32) (B) Refer the patient for speech consultation.

For individuals who are receiving enteral nutrition and have difficulty swallowing, a speech therapist can provide exercises and techniques to improve swallowing function and reduce the risk of aspiration. This is an important step in ensuring patients are able to receive the necessary nutrition to support their health.

(33) (D) Refer the patient to a registered dietitian for dietary consultation.

A registered dietitian can provide guidance on the composition of the enteral nutrition the patient is receiving and make recommendations for adjustments based on the patient's nutritional needs and medical conditions.

(34) (C) Infections, such as a cold or the flu.

Infections, such as a cold or the flu, are not commonly associated with the need for alternate forms of nutrition administration. Alternate forms of nutrition administration are typically used in medical conditions or scenarios where a patient is unable to obtain adequate nutrition through oral intake alone.

(35) (B) The patient's needs and preferences.

Patient-centered care is an approach to health care that prioritizes the patient's needs, preferences and values. It places the patient, rather than the health care provider or the medical treatment plan, at the center of care.

(36) (B) Prioritizing the patient's unique needs, values and cultural background.

To prioritize the patient's unique needs, values and cultural background. Individualized care is a holistic approach that prioritizes each patient's unique needs. It involves considering the patient's values, preferences and cultural background and tailoring care to meet those needs.

(37) (C) 20 seconds.

The recommended duration for hand hygiene using an alcohol-based hand sanitizer is at least 20 seconds. This duration ensures proper coverage and effective killing of microorganisms on the hands.

(38) (B) Change the dressing immediately using sterile technique.

If a central line dressing becomes loose or soiled, it should be changed immediately using a sterile technique to minimize the risk of infection. A loose or soiled dressing can allow bacteria to enter the site and potentially cause a serious infection such as a bloodstream infection.

(39) (B) Using a 10 ml or larger syringe

To prevent damage to the central line, a 10ml or larger syringe should be used when flushing the line. Smaller syringes can create too much pressure, which could damage the line and increase the risk of infection. Clean technique is important, but sterile technique is typically recommended when handling a central line. Tap water should not be used because it's not sterile and flushing frequency depends on the healthcare provider's instructions and the type of central line.

(40) (A) To create an atmosphere that is conducive to effective communication.

The environment plays a significant role in communication, as factors such as temperature, lighting, noise and privacy can affect the patient's comfort level. This can make it difficult for the patient to focus on communication and can also lead to nonverbal cues of discomfort.

(41) (C) Not asking patients to clarify their statements if there is something not understood.

If a health care professional does not understand something a patient has said, it is important to ask for clarification in order to have a full understanding of the patient's needs and preferences. This can help to ensure effective communication and build trust with the patient.

(42) (C) Include the daughter in all aspects of the patient's care, including decision-making, but ensure that the health care team is consulted and informed about any changes.

This option allows for active involvement and support from the daughter while also ensuring that the health care team is informed and involved in decision-making and treatment planning. It balances the daughter's desire to be involved and provide support with the need for professional medical care and guidance.

(43) (B) Specific, measurable and achievable.

These goals are set for patients with the goal of improving their health and well-being and should be collaboratively developed with the patient.

(44) (D) To take medications as prescribed.

Taking medications as prescribed is a specific and measurable aspect of the health goal, as the health care provider can directly monitor it. This action can also lead to the achievement of the goal of reducing blood sugar levels to within normal range. Improving physical activity, reducing stress and eating a healthy diet are also important factors in managing diabetes, but they may not be directly related to achieving this specific health goal.

(45) (C) Technological advancement.

The ANA guidelines for patient-centered care include respect for patient autonomy, partnership with patients and families, compassionate care, coordination of care, cultural sensitivity, continuity of care and patient and family education, but not technological advancement.

(46) (A) Providing care that is consistent over time and across different settings.

Continuity of care refers to the provision of care that is consistent and not interrupted, regardless of changes in time or location of care. This is an important aspect of patient-centered care, as it helps ensure that the patient receives comprehensive and coordinated care.

(47) (C) It emphasizes the importance of respecting the patients' right to make decisions about their own care.

This principle is important in patient-centered care, as it recognizes the patient's autonomy and self-determination and ensures that the patient's preferences and values are taken into consideration when making decisions about their care.

(48) (A) To help them take an active role in their own care and feel more in control of their health.

The objective of providing personalized resources to patients is to help them take an active role in their own care and feel more in control of their health. This is achieved by evaluating what resources best meet their individual needs, which can involve assessing their medical history, current health status and personal preferences.

(49) (A) By assessing their medical history and individual preferences.

The process of providing personalized resources to patients involves evaluating what resources best meet their individual needs by assessing their medical history and individual preferences. This can help patients take an active role in their own care and feel more in control of their health. Personalized resources can be provided in various ways, such as through brochures, pamphlets, videos or online resources. Patients can also be directed to outside organizations or agencies that provide additional resources and support.

(50) (A) To evaluate the performance of individual providers.

Measuring patient satisfaction is a way to gather feedback from patients and assess the quality of care provided by a health care facility or provider. By analyzing patient satisfaction data, health care organizations can identify areas for improvement and evaluate the performance of individual providers.

(51) (D) It must comply with state-specific guidelines and regulations.

For an advance directive to be considered legally binding, it must comply with state-specific guidelines and regulations.

This means that the document must be created and executed in accordance with the laws and regulations of the state in which the individual resides. The requirement for physician approval in the event of a terminal illness or injury does not apply to advance directives.

(52) (B) Living will.

Based on the scenario, the most likely document is a living will. A living will outlines an individual's preferences for medical treatment and end-of-life care in the event they become incapacitated and unable to communicate. In this case, if the patient becomes unable to make decisions or communicate her wishes, her living will should help guide her medical team in providing the appropriate level of care and treatment.

(53) (B) Physician's directive.

In this case, the patient has a document in place outlining his end-of-life preferences, which would help ensure that his wishes are honored in the event of a medical emergency. The document he has is most likely a physician's directive. A physician's directive is a written statement that specifies an individual's desire to forgo life-sustaining treatments in the event of a terminal illness or injury.

(54) (D) Health care power of attorney.

In this case, the health care team is looking for guidance on how to proceed with medical treatment, as the patient is unable to make decisions due to a stroke. The most useful document in this situation would be a health care power of attorney. A health care power of attorney is a document that designates a trusted individual to make health care decisions on behalf of the patient in the event they become incapacitated.

(55) (C) Refrain from performing CPR but seek clarification from Mr. Patel's family or health care proxy.

Although Mr. Patel has a DNR tattoo, health care providers should always seek clarification from the patient's family or health care proxy, as tattoos are not legally recognized as valid advance directives.

(56) (A) Adherence to cultural customs.

Different cultures have different customs, and it is important to respect them and make the preparation process as dignified and appropriate as possible. In addition, state laws and agency policies must also be followed to ensure the proper preparation and handling of the body.

(57) (B) Only in some cultures and circumstances.

It may be important to allow the family to prepare or assist in preparing the body, taking into consideration cultural customs, state laws and agency policies and procedures.

(58) (C) State laws and agency policies and procedures.

In the event of an unexpected or unanticipated death, the preparation of the body for viewing or release to a funeral home is guided by state laws and agency policies and procedures to ensure compliance with all relevant regulations.

(59) (B) Pre-death declaration.

The process of a person deciding before death to donate their organs or provide anatomic gifts is called an advance directive or pre-death declaration. This allows individuals to make informed decisions about their health care, including the donation of their organs, before they become unable to communicate their wishes.

(60) (A) By carrying a donor card or by indicating her preference on her driver's license.

Some individuals choose to carry a donor card to clearly express their willingness to donate their organs or tissues. In some states, individuals can also indicate their preference to donate on their driver's license. This makes it easier for their family and medical team to follow their wishes.

(61) (A) To coordinate with the organ-sharing network.

The immediate notification of the physician is an important step in the organ and tissue donation process. This allows for the proper handling and preservation of the donated organs and tissues and ensures that the donation is made in a lawful and ethical manner that respects the wishes of the individual and their family.

(62) (D) Encourage Mr. Alessio to make a decision regarding organ donation.

Since Mr. Alessio has not yet indicated his wishes regarding organ donation, it would be appropriate for the medical team to encourage him to make a decision. This allows Mr. Alessio to make an informed choice about his end-of-life preferences and ensures that his wishes are respected.

(63) (C) Transfer Mrs. Green to hospice care and respect her wishes regarding dialysis.

Mrs. Green has expressed that she does not want to undergo dialysis and has indicated that she would like to be placed in hospice care. The medical team should respect her wishes and transfer her to hospice care. Notifying the organ-sharing network and beginning the process of obtaining family permission for organ donation is also important, but it is not the most immediate step to take.

(64) (B) Assess the patient's motor function and sensory level regularly

For patients receiving medication through an epidural catheter, a key assessment is regular monitoring of motor function and sensory level. This can help to identify any potential complications like epidural hematoma or abscess which can lead to serious neurological consequences if not detected early.

(65) (C) Position the patient in a supine position and notify the healthcare provider

A severe headache following the removal of an epidural catheter could indicate a post-dural puncture headache (PDPH), which is caused by leakage of cerebrospinal fluid (CSF) from the puncture site. This is considered a medical emergency.

(66) (B) It allows for lower doses of individual medications, reducing the risk of side effects

Multimodal pain management involves the use of multiple different types of pain relief measures, both pharmacologic and non-pharmacologic. The primary advantage of this approach is that it allows for the use of lower doses of individual medications, which can reduce the risk of side effects and potential complications associated with higher doses of a single medication.

(67) (B) Administration of acetaminophen, gabapentin, and the use of a patient-controlled analgesia (PCA) pump with morphine

Multimodal pain management involves the use of different types of pain relief measures, including pharmacologic agents with different mechanisms of action and potentially also non-pharmacologic interventions.

(68) (B) When pain appears to be related to pressure or poor body alignment

Repositioning can be an effective non-pharmacological intervention for managing pain that is related to pressure, poor body alignment, or immobility. Repositioning can alleviate pressure points, improve circulation, and contribute to comfort.

(69) (C) Applying a cold pack to the ankle

For acute injuries like sprains, applying cold can help to reduce swelling and numb the area, decreasing pain. Cold should be applied for 15-20 minutes at a time, with breaks in between to prevent damage to the skin. Heat can increase swelling in acute injuries, so it's typically not recommended in the first 24-48 hours following the injury.

(70) (C) Acupuncture can be a beneficial complement to traditional pain management strategies for some patients

Acupuncture, a practice originating from traditional Chinese medicine, involves the insertion of very thin needles through the skin at strategic points on the body. While the exact mechanisms are not fully understood, it is thought to stimulate nerves, muscles, and connective tissue to increase blood flow and stimulate the body's natural painkillers.

(71) (A) Ensure the acupuncturist is licensed and follows safe, clean needle practices

For a patient considering acupuncture, it is important to ensure the acupuncturist is licensed and follows safe practices, including the use of sterile, single-use needles. This helps to prevent complications such as infections. Self-acupuncture is not recommended due to the risk of injury or improper technique. Acupuncture may be used in conjunction with other pain management strategies and should not necessarily replace them.

(72) (C) Aromatherapy may provide subjective relief of mild symptoms of anxiety for some individuals.

Aromatherapy, which involves the use of essential oils, may provide subjective relief of mild symptoms of anxiety for some individuals. However, while some studies suggest potential benefits, more comprehensive research is needed. Aromatherapy is not considered a primary or standalone treatment for serious psychiatric conditions but can be a complementary therapy.

(73) (C) Some patients may have allergic reactions to certain essential oils.

When considering the use of aromatherapy, it's important to remember that some patients may have allergic reactions to certain essential oils. Additionally, some oils can cause skin irritation if applied undiluted, and many are not safe for ingestion.

(74) (D) Burial or cremation permits.

In order to bury or cremate the deceased, a permit must be obtained from the local government. This permit is an important legal requirement and must be obtained before any funeral arrangements can take place.

(75) (B) After the death is reported to the authorities.

A death certificate must be completed by a physician or coroner and includes information, such as the cause of death, time of death and the deceased's personal details. This document is a necessary step in the process of reporting a death, but it is typically obtained after the death has been reported to the appropriate authorities, such as the local police or coroner's office.

(76) (C) To provide official documentation of the cause, time and the deceased's personal details.

A death certificate must be completed by a physician or coroner, who includes information, such as the cause of death, time of death and the deceased's personal details. This document serves as a permanent record of the death and is required for various legal, financial and personal purposes.

(77) (B) Cisplatin.

Cisplatin is a chemotherapy medication that has been shown to cause side effects, such as nausea, vomiting and loss of appetite. These side effects can contribute to malnutrition by decreasing appetite and nutrient absorption.

(78) (A) Clear liquid diet.

Clear liquid diets are low residue and consist of water, broth, clear juices, tea and soda. These diets are used for a short period, as they provide inadequate nutrition for long-term use.

(79) (D) To identify the patient's goals and expected outcomes, as well as steps to achieve them.

The outcome/goal statements provide a clear, concise description of what patients hope to achieve from the care they receive. The nurse uses this information to determine appropriate nursing interventions and create a plan of care that will help patients reach their goals.

(80) (C) To deliver care to the patient.

The implementation phase is the time when the nurse carries out the care plan and provides care to the patient. The nurse's primary responsibility during this phase is to deliver the care that has been determined necessary to meet the patient's needs.

(81) (A) To determine if the patient's goals have been met.

The evaluation phase is the time when the nurse assesses the outcomes of the care provided to the patient. The main objective of this evaluation is to determine if the care plan was effective in meeting the patient's needs and achieving the individual's goals.

(82) (A) To gather as much information as possible about the patient's health status and needs.

The information gathered is used to identify the patient's strengths, weaknesses and areas of concern and make appropriate nursing diagnoses, formulate outcome/goal statements, determine nursing interventions and evaluate the patient's progress.

(83) (B) Stop the flush and assess the patient and the device

Pain during a saline flush could indicate a problem with the portacath, such as a blockage, infection, or mechanical issue. It could also potentially indicate that the needle is not properly positioned in the septum of the port. The nurse should immediately stop the flush and assess both the patient and the device. If necessary, the healthcare provider or an appropriate specialist should be contacted.

(84) (B) The portacath needs to be accessed using a non-coring (Huber) needle

A portacath, a type of central venous catheter, can be used for the administration of IV contrast during a CT scan. However, it should be accessed using a non-coring (Huber) needle, which is designed to prevent damage to the port septum. The portacath does not need to be removed for the procedure, and prophylactic antibiotics are not typically necessary just for contrast administration. As always, the radiology department and the patient's healthcare provider should be consulted for any specific requirements or precautions.

(85) (B) Completing a thorough health and medical history.

During the assessment phase, the nurse's main focus is to gather as much information as possible about the patient's health status and needs, and the first step in this process is to gather a comprehensive health and medical history. This includes information about the patient's past and present medical conditions, medications, allergies and family history, which can help provide important context for the chest pain.

(86) (B) The patient's health and medical history.

This subjective information is obtained through verbal communication with the patient and provides insight into the patient's experiences, feelings and perceptions about health and well-being.

(87) (B) The process of making an appropriate diagnosis.

Clinical reasoning is the process of thoroughly analyzing information, recognizing cues, sorting and organizing the data and determining a patient's strengths and unmet needs in order to make an appropriate diagnosis.

(88) (C) To organize and communicate assessment findings.

The PES system is a structured method used to succinctly identify a patient's needs and concerns and help nurses organize and communicate their assessment findings in a clear and consistent manner.

(89) (C) Problem.

The first element of the PES system is P (problem), which is a brief nursing diagnosis label that represents a pattern of related cues sourced from the official NANDA-I list.

(90) (B) The underlying cause or contributor to the problem.

The etiology element of the PES system is represented by the "related to" phrase or etiology and represents the underlying cause or contributor to the problem.

(91) (D) All of the above.

In the process of identifying patterns and symptoms in nursing assessments, a nurse must follow a systematic approach, which includes asking questions, validating information and analyzing symptoms; highlighting important symptoms, creating a list of symptoms and clustering together similar symptoms; analyzing and interpreting symptoms; and selecting a suitable nursing diagnosis label from the NANDA-I list.

(92) (C) Analyze and interpret the symptoms of chest pain and shortness of breath.

After identifying and highlighting important symptoms during the assessment process, the next step is to analyze and interpret those symptoms to understand what they signify or represent when they occur together. In this case, the symptoms of chest pain and shortness of breath may be indicative of angina or a heart attack and will require further analysis in order to arrive at a nursing diagnosis label from the NANDA-I list.

(93) (C) To address life-threatening needs first.

The patient's immediate needs, such as airway, breathing and circulation, should be considered first.

(94) (B) By addressing the patient's physiological needs first.

Maslow's hierarchy of needs starts with the most basic needs, such as physiological needs, before moving on to higher-level needs.

(95) (B) ABC approach and Maslow's hierarchy of needs.

In the planning phase, it is important to prioritize the patient's immediate needs first (using the ABC approach) and consider Maslow's hierarchy of needs to ensure that life-threatening needs are addressed first. This information, along with the patient's history and assessment findings, is used to determine appropriate patient-specific outcomes and interventions.

(96) (B) Managing symptoms.

The main focus of the implementation phase of the nursing process is to manage symptoms and provide support and assistance to the patient and the family, helping them function at their highest level possible.

(97) (C) Carrying out individualized interventions.

The nurse plays a crucial role during the implementation phase of the nursing process by carrying out individualized interventions that have been tailored to the patient's specific needs. Option A, writing the care plan, and Option B, monitoring the patient's progress, are important aspects of the nursing process but take place in different stages.

(98) (B) To protect the facility and nurse in case of legal dispute.

Keeping accurate and detailed records of nursing interventions and patient outcomes is crucial for protecting the facility and the nurse in case of a legal dispute. Proper documentation serves as evidence of the actions taken and provides a clear and concise record of what was done and what outcomes were achieved.

(99) (A) To evaluate care and patient outcomes as part of charting.

Problem-oriented charting involves evaluating care and patient outcomes as part of charting and is often used in many facilities. This type of charting helps the nurse focus on the problem at hand and assess the effectiveness of the interventions in resolving it.

(100) (C) To reassess patients and compare their condition before and after the interventions.

Evaluation is an ongoing aspect. It involves reassessing patients and comparing their conditions before and after the interventions. The nurse's assessment of a patient's response to interventions is valuable in determining if adjustments need to be made to the care plan.

(101) (A) To provide feedback and identify areas for improvement.

This helps health care professionals understand the strengths and weaknesses of their documentation practices and provides an opportunity for them to improve their practices and meet the necessary standards and requirements.

(102) (B) To document patient care in a clear, concise and accurate manner.

This includes training on how to navigate the technology and equipment, enter data and retrieve information, as well as how to use the technology and equipment to document patient care in a manner that meets the necessary standards and requirements.

(103) (D) All of the above.

Health care professionals should be familiar with a variety of aspects of technology and equipment use, including how to document patient care in a clear, concise and accurate manner; the features and capabilities of the technology and equipment; and how to navigate the system and enter data.

(104) (B) Surgical site infection (SSI) after an elective surgery

Healthcare-associated infections (HAIs) are infections that patients acquire while receiving healthcare treatment. Surgical site infections (SSIs) are a common type of HAI that occur after surgery, specifically at the site of the surgical incision.

(105) (D) All of the above.

Health care professionals should be familiar with a variety of aspects related to troubleshooting technology and equipment problems, including the contact information for technical support, the troubleshooting procedures for the technology and equipment they are using and how to reach out for assistance when needed.

(106) (C) To quickly and effectively resolve problems.

Knowing how to reach out for technical support when troubleshooting technology and equipment problems is beneficial because it allows health care professionals to quickly and effectively resolve any problems that may arise.

(107) (B) Records that are becoming increasingly popular in providing real-time access to patient information.

Electronic health records are digital versions of a patient's medical history, which can include medical test results, prescription details and other health information. By providing real-time access to patient information, EHRs can help improve communication and continuity of care and reduce medical errors.

(108) (B) To provide remote health care services, such as telemedicine, teleconsultation and remote patient monitoring.

Telehealth is the use of technology to provide remote health care services, such as telemedicine, teleconsultation and remote patient monitoring.

(109) (B) AI is used to improve the accuracy and speed of diagnoses, support decision-making and automate routine tasks.

Artificial intelligence is being used in health care to improve the accuracy and speed of diagnoses, as well as to support decision-making and automate routine tasks. This can help health care providers deliver better care while also freeing up time for other important tasks.

(110) (B) IoT is used in health care to connect medical devices and enable the collection and analysis of real-time patient data, allowing health care providers to make more informed decisions.

In health care, IoT devices—such as medical devices, wearables and sensors—can be used to collect and transmit real-time patient data, which health care providers can then analyze to make more informed decisions and improve patient care.

(111) (A) To perform surgeries and assist in patient care, including rehabilitation and physical therapy.

The use of robotics in health care can help improve patient outcomes and increase efficiency by freeing health care professionals to focus on more complex tasks and providing patients with more personalized care.

(112) (A) The combination of nursing science, computer science and information science that focuses on the use of technology and information to improve patient care.

Nursing informatics encompasses areas such as EHRs and other health information systems, data analysis and decision-making, education and training, research and standards and regulations.

(113) (B) Ensuring the use of technology and information systems in patient care complies with relevant standards and regulations.

Other nursing informatics responsibilities include conducting research, analyzing data, educating and training health care professionals and working with EHRs and other health information systems.

(114) (B) Supervising staff and managing specific units or departments.

The charge nurse is a higher-level position in the nursing chain of command and is responsible for supervising staff and managing specific units or departments. Charge nurses oversee the day-to-day operations of the unit and make sure patient care is delivered effectively and efficiently.

(115) (B) A hierarchy of leadership and authority within the nursing profession.

The chain of command in nursing refers to the hierarchy of leadership and authority within the nursing profession, establishing a clear line of communication and accountability, ensuring that decisions are made at the appropriate level and everyone knows who to report to and who to contact if they have any issues or concerns.

(116) (D) Nurse technicians and staff nurses.

The chain of command in nursing typically starts with entry-level positions, such as nurse technicians and staff nurses, who are responsible for providing direct patient care. It then progresses to higher-level positions—such as charge nurses, nursing managers and directors—who are responsible for supervising staff and managing specific units or departments.

(117) (B) To ensure that decisions are made at the appropriate level.

The main purpose of the chain of command in nursing is to establish a clear line of communication and accountability, ensuring that decisions are made at the appropriate level. This helps ensure that everyone knows who to report to and who to contact if they have any issues or concerns.

(118) (B) Providing direct patient care.

Entry-level positions in the nursing chain of command, such as nurse technicians and staff nurses, are responsible for providing direct patient care. The higher-level positions—such as charge nurses, nursing managers and directors—are responsible for supervising staff and managing specific units or departments.

(119) (C) A communication skill that involves paying attention and understanding the message.

Active listening in nursing is a communication skill that involves paying attention to what others are saying, understanding their message and providing an appropriate response. It helps the nurse understand the patient's needs and experiences, leading to improved patient outcomes.

(120) (D) All of the above.

The benefits of using active listening techniques in nursing include improved patient outcomes, the opportunity for the nurse to clarify any confusion and a deeper understanding of the patient's needs and experiences.

(121) (D) All of the above.

Some active listening techniques that nurses can use include observing the speaker's behavior and body language, repeating back the main point or message, clarifying anything that is unclear and reserving judgment. These techniques help the nurse understand the patient's message and avoid misunderstandings.

(122) (B) To provide high-quality health service.

Verbal communication is an essential skill for nurses in providing high-quality health service. Nurses must be able to communicate effectively with patients and other health care professionals by speaking clearly, accurately and honestly.

(123) (D) All of the above.

To achieve excellent verbal communication in nursing, it is important to consider factors such as speaking with clarity and accuracy, understanding the audience's background, being aware of the tone of voice, encouraging patients to communicate, avoiding condescending pet names and speaking in clear, complete sentences.

(124) (C) Asking open-ended questions.

By asking open-ended questions—such as "Can you tell me a bit more about that?"—nurses can encourage patients to share their thoughts and feelings. This helps the nurse understand the patient's perspective and provide better care.

(125) (B) To create a rapport with patients and build trust.

Nonverbal communication is as important as verbal communication in creating a rapport with patients and building trust. As a nurse, it is important to be aware of the nonverbal cues you are sending and use them to create a positive and empathetic connection with patients.

(126) (C) Maintain eye contact and nod your head.

Maintaining eye contact and nodding while patients are speaking is an effective way to show interest in nonverbal communication. A simple smile can also go a long way in creating a positive and welcoming environment for patients.

(127) (C) Using an open posture.

Avoiding prolonged staring, sitting down and leaning forward when interacting with patients and using open posture are examples of effective nonverbal communication techniques. On the other hand, crossing arms or legs and using threatening body language can convey defensiveness or closed-mindedness, which is not appropriate in a health care setting.

(128) (B) To record accurate and legible patient medical records.

The primary purpose of written communication skills for nurses is to record accurate and legible patient medical records. Other health care professionals use these records to provide the best possible care to patients.

(129) (D) Take notes immediately and write legibly and clearly.

To improve their written communication skills, nurses should take notes immediately and write legibly and clearly. This will help ensure that important information is not forgotten and that the writing is easy to read and understand.

(130) (C) Accuracy of information.

Other health care professionals use the records to provide the best possible care to patients, so it is essential that they be accurate, current and written in a clear and legible manner.

(131) (C) Active listening.

The first step in effective conflict resolution in nursing is active listening. By listening actively, nurses can understand the perspectives of all parties involved and identify the underlying issues that are causing the conflict.

(132) (A) Neutral third parties.

Nurses can help resolve conflicts or disputes between patients and health care staff by acting as mediators and neutral third parties.

(133) (C) Active listening.

By actively listening to both parties, the nurse can understand their perspectives and identify the underlying issues causing the conflict. Then, using communication, empathy and problem-solving skills, the nurse can help resolve the conflict in a respectful and effective manner.

(134) (D) All of the above.

By understanding and sharing the patient's feelings, actively listening to their concerns and being sensitive to their cultural background, the nurse can help defuse tensions and resolve the conflict in a respectful and effective manner.

(135) (D) All of the above.

The purpose of the SBAR tool in health care communication is to reduce the risk of errors, focus on the most important information and improve coordination of care. The SBAR tool provides a clear and concise way to communicate important patient information, ensuring that all relevant information is communicated and follow-up actions are taken in a timely manner.

(136) (C) A description of the patient's current condition.

The Assessment section of the SBAR tool includes a description of the patient's current condition, such as vital signs, symptoms and any changes in their condition.

(137) (A) To transfer patient care from one health care professional to another.

Hand-off refers to the process of transferring patient care from one health care professional to another. It is important that hand-offs be done in a clear and organized manner to ensure that all relevant patient information is passed on and that continuity of care is maintained.

(138) (A) Closed-loop communication involves repeating the information provided, while check-back specifically refers to the act of following up with the person who provided the information.

Closed-loop communication is a larger process that encompasses multiple steps, such as repeating the information, giving feedback and confirming that the information was acted upon. Check-back is a specific step within the closed-loop communication process.

(139) (C) Verbal intervention.

Verbal intervention involves using calm and measured language to diffuse a situation. This can include using a calm tone of voice, speaking slowly and avoiding confrontational language. It is an effective way to defuse tensions and build rapport with the patient, helping keep everyone safe.

(140) (B) To prioritize care based on patients' conditions and potential risks.

The objective is to ensure that the most critical patient needs are met and to provide the best possible care for patients.

(141) (D) All of the above.

The Modified Early Warning Score (MEWS) uses a combination of vital signs, patient history and lab results to identify patients at risk of deterioration. The National Early Warning Score (NEWS) uses similar parameters as MEWS but with a different scoring system. The Rapid Response Team (RRT) is activated when a patient's condition deteriorates and requires immediate medical attention.

(142) (D) Self-regulation, problem-solving, analysis, interpretation and inference.

Critical thinking in health care involves several key elements, including the ability to monitor one's own thinking (self-regulation), identify and analyze problems (problem-solving), break down information (analysis), understand the meaning of information (interpretation) and draw conclusions based on evidence (inference).

(143) (D) All of the above.

Workplace safety in health care is concerned with protecting nurses from physical injuries and accidents, emotional and psychological stress and hazards in the physical environment. This includes implementing proper ergonomics, providing PPE, promoting a positive work environment, ensuring proper ventilation and lighting and controlling temperature and humidity.

(144) (B) Providing opportunities for self-care and stress management, such as exercise and meditation.

Encouraging nurses to take regular breaks throughout the workday, fostering a supportive work environment and providing mental health services are all important aspects, but providing opportunities for self-care and stress management is the primary strategy.

(145) (A) Physical and emotional exhaustion.

Burnout is a state of physical and emotional exhaustion, depersonalization and reduced personal accomplishment that can occur as a result of prolonged stress and high demands, leading to feelings of detachment, cynicism and a sense of failure.

(146) (B) The allocation of staffing.

Resource allocation in health care organizations is mainly focused on determining how staffing resources will be distributed and used within the organization. Adequate staffing is critical for ensuring safe and high-quality care, and the allocation of staffing can have a significant impact on the quality of care provided to patients and the well-being of health care workers.

(147) (D) All of the above.

These elements cover various aspects of ethical practices in nursing, including ethical decision-making, adherence to legal and regulatory requirements, respect for patient rights, promotion of an ethical work environment and professional development.

(148) (B) Provide accurate and complete information about medical history and current health status.

One of the responsibilities of a patient in terms of health care is to provide accurate and complete information about the person's medical history and current health status. This information helps health care providers make informed decisions about the patient's care and treatment.

(149) (D) All of the above.

The AMSN's standards of practice for medical-surgical nurses encompass all of the components listed in the question, including assessment, diagnosis, outcomes identification, planning, implementation, evaluation, professional practice, education and leadership.

(150) (C) Formulating research questions or hypotheses.

In the fifth step of the quantitative research process, the researcher defines clear research questions or hypotheses that guide the study and can be tested. This step is important for ensuring the focus and direction of the research and for allowing for the testing of specific relationships between variables.

Test 2: Questions

(1) What is the definition of polypharmacy?

(A) The use of a single medication

(B) The use of multiple medications

(C) The use of unnecessary or inappropriate medications

(D) The use of herbal products or supplements

(2) Which population is particularly at risk for polypharmacy?

(A) Children

(B) Older adults

(C) Patients with mental illnesses

(D) All of the above

(3) A patient has been taking multiple medications for a chronic condition, but the health care provider notices that the patient is experiencing adverse reactions and medication interactions. Which step can the health care provider take to minimize the risks associated with polypharmacy in this case?

(A) Increase the frequency of the patient's medication regimen.

(B) Modify the patient's medication regimen by substituting certain medications.

(C) Regularly review the patient's medication list and adjust or reduce the number of medications as necessary.

(D) Maintain the current medication regimen and monitor the patient's progress.

(4) What is the goal of regular medication reviews in drug stewardship?

(A) To identify potential issues in a patient's medication list

(B) To monitor for adverse reactions to medications

(C) To ensure patients are taking their medications correctly

(D) To compare a patient's medication list to the medications prescribed

(5) What are the potential consequences of improper medication disposal?

(A) Financial penalties for health care providers

(B) Contamination of the water supply and harm to wildlife

(C) Adverse reactions in patients

(D) Medication errors and increased health care costs

(6) What is the first step in developing an effective treatment plan for pain management?

(A) Assessing pain

(B) Prescribing medication

(C) Referring to a specialist

(D) Conducting a physical examination

(7) Pain is classified _____.

(A) As either acute or chronic

(B) As either mild or severe

(C) As either physical or emotional

(D) As either short term or long term

(8) A patient is experiencing pain, and the health care provider has used the 0-10 rating scale to assess the pain. The patient's score is 8. What should the health care provider do next?

(A) Prescribe a strong pain medication.

(B) Refer the patient to a specialist.

(C) Assess the patient's pain again in a few hours.

(D) Develop a pain management plan that includes a combination of medication and nonmedication options.

(9) Which types of medications are typically used for acute pain management?

(A) Antidepressants, anticonvulsants and muscle relaxants

(B) Nonsteroidal anti-inflammatory drugs (NSAIDs), acetaminophen and opioid analgesics

(C) Transcutaneous electrical nerve stimulation (TENS) and spinal cord stimulation

(D) Physical therapy, cognitive-behavioral therapy and occupational therapy

(10) Which nonpharmacologic interventions are commonly used in chronic pain management?

(A) Antidepressants, anticonvulsants and muscle relaxants

(B) NSAIDs, acetaminophen and opioid analgesics

(C) TENS and spinal cord stimulation

(D) Physical therapy, cognitive-behavioral therapy and occupational therapy

(11) What is the typical incubation period for the flu after exposure?

(A) 1-4 days

(B) 1-2 weeks

(C) 3-4 weeks

(D) 6-8 weeks

(12) A patient with chronic pain is prescribed a medication by the physician. The patient has been taking the medication for several weeks but has not reported any significant improvement in pain. The nurse should _____.

(A) Increase the dosage of the medication without consulting the physician.

(B) Advise the patient to continue taking the medication as prescribed and inform the physician of the lack of improvement.

(C) Suggest alternative pain management methods, such as physical therapy or cognitive-behavioral therapy, to the patient and inform the physician.

(D) Stop the medication without consulting the physician.

(13) What is the main benefit of a multimodal approach to pain management?

(A) Reduced risk of side effects

(B) Targeting multiple pain pathways

(C) Improved pain control

(D) All of the above

(14) A patient has just been discharged from the hospital and is experiencing pain in his incision site. The nurse should do which of the following to ensure that the patient's expectation of effective pain relief is met?

(A) Administer a pain medication and reassess the patient's pain in one hour.

(B) Wait for the patient to request pain medication and only administer it if he asks.

(C) Assess the patient's pain using a validated pain assessment tool, document the results and administer medication per the physician's order.

(D) Advise the patient to take over-the-counter pain medication as needed.

(15) A patient is experiencing pain, and the nurse notices that she is uncomfortable discussing her pain. What should the nurse do to ensure that the patient's rights and well-being are being promoted?

(A) Ignore the patient's discomfort and continue to ask about her pain.

(B) Respect the patient's discomfort and suggest alternative methods for communicating about her pain.

(C) Assume the patient is not in pain and refrain from administering any pain medication.

(D) Encourage the patient to "tough it out" and not discuss her pain.

(16) A patient has a specific cultural belief about pain management that conflicts with the treatment plan. What should the nurse do to ensure that the patient's rights and well-being are being promoted?

(A) Ignore the patient's cultural beliefs and continue with the treatment plan.

(B) Inform the patient that his cultural belief is incorrect and that the treatment plan is the only option.

(C) Discuss the patient's cultural beliefs with the interdisciplinary team and work to develop a culturally sensitive treatment plan.

(D) Advise the patient to ignore his cultural belief and follow the treatment plan.

(17) A patient is experiencing pain, and the nurse is unsure of what nonpharmacological pain management method to use. What should the patient do to ensure that the patient's needs are being met?

(A) Choose a nonpharmacological pain management method at random.

(B) Ignore the patient's pain and not implement any nonpharmacological pain management methods.

(C) Consult with other members of the health care team, including pain specialists and physical therapists, to determine the most appropriate nonpharmacological pain management method.

(D) Advise the patient to continue with the current treatment plan and not explore nonpharmacological options.

(18) What is the purpose of cutaneous stimulation as a CAM method for pain management?

(A) To channel healing energy to the patient

(B) To stimulate the skin and underlying tissues to alleviate pain and improve circulation

(C) To balance the flow of energy and alleviate pain

(D) To control certain physiological processes

(19) How does acupuncture work as a CAM method for pain management?

(A) By channeling healing energy to the patient

(B) By stimulating the skin and underlying tissues

(C) By inserting needles into special points on the body to balance the flow of energy and alleviate pain

(D) By providing feedback on the physiological state

(20) What is the focus of cognitive and behavioral pain management as a CAM method?

(A) Channeling healing energy to the patient

(B) Stimulating the skin and underlying tissues

(C) Inserting needles into special points on the body

(D) Using techniques such as relaxation, visualization and mindfulness to manage pain

(21) How does biofeedback work as a CAM method for pain management?

(A) By channeling healing energy to the patient

(B) By stimulating the skin and underlying tissues

(C) By inserting needles into special points on the body

(D) By enabling an individual to control certain physiological processes to manage pain and other symptoms

(22) How does aromatherapy work as a CAM method for pain management?

(A) By channeling healing energy to the patient

(B) By stimulating the skin and underlying tissues

(C) By inserting needles into special points on the body

(D) By using essential oils from plants to promote physical and psychological well-being by stimulating the olfactory system and activating certain areas of the brain

(23) What is the purpose of obtaining informed consent from a patient before a surgical procedure?

(A) To document the patient's understanding and agreement to the procedure

(B) To ensure the correct patient, procedure and site are being worked on

(C) To monitor the patient's vital signs before, during and after the procedure

(D) To prepare the patient for surgery by positioning him in the correct position

(24) What is the purpose of a time-out in a surgical procedure?

(A) To obtain informed consent from the patient

(B) To ensure the correct patient, procedure and site are being worked on

(C) To monitor the patient's vital signs before, during and after the procedure

(D) To prepare patients for surgery by positioning them in the correct position

(25) What is the importance of monitoring the patient's vital signs before, during and after a surgical procedure?

(A) To obtain informed consent from the patient

(B) To ensure the correct patient, procedure and site are being worked on

(C) To monitor patients' well-being and ensure that they are stable

(D) To prepare patients for surgery by positioning them in the correct position

(26) What is the primary use of cefazolin (Ancef) as a medication?

(A) To reduce oral and respiratory secretions

(B) To induce sedation, anxiety and amnesic effects

(C) To prevent postoperative infection

(D) To stabilize blood glucose

(27) What is the main function of famotidine (Pepcid) as a medication?

(A) To help the patient become more active

(B) To decrease happiness hormones

(C) To increase happiness hormones

(D) To reduce acid secretion and gastric volume

(28) What is the primary use of atropine (Isopto Atropine) as a medication?

(A) To help the patient go to sleep easily

(B) To help with an upset stomach

(C) To reduce oral and respiratory secretions

(D) To induce relaxation

(29) What is the main function of midazolam (Versed) as a medication?

(A) To relieve pain during preoperative procedures

(B) To promote gastric emptying and prevent nausea and vomiting

(C) To induce sedation, anxiety and amnesic effects

(D) To manage hypertension

(30) What is the primary purpose of the post-anesthesia care unit (PACU)?

(A) To provide close monitoring and care for patients immediately after surgery

(B) To ensure that patients receive the care they need in a timely manner

(C) To provide easy access to anesthesia and OR personnel

(D) All of the above

(31) A patient is experiencing severe pain after surgery, and the nurse is unsure of how to properly manage it. What is the most appropriate method of pain management for a patient in the PACU?

(A) Administering an NSAID

(B) Administering an opioid medication

(C) Utilizing heat therapy or cold therapy

(D) Implementing a combination of pharmacological and nonpharmacological pain management methods

(32) What is the first step in post-surgery patient care?

(A) Evaluating the patient's body temperature and capillary refill

(B) Assessing the patient's level of consciousness and orientation

(C) Assessing the patient's ABC status

(D) Implementing postoperative orders related to incision care

(33) What is a useful tool for monitoring oxygenation in a patient after surgery?

(A) Capnography

(B) Pulse oximetry

(C) Electrocardiography

(D) Blood pressure measurement

(34) Which of the following is important to check for in patients who have received a regional anesthetic?

(A) Residual sensory or motor blockade

(B) Fluid balance in the urinary system

(C) Incision care and management of dressings or drainage

(D) All of the above

(35) Which of the following should be included in the assessment of a patient's urinary system after surgery?

(A) Input and output measurements

(B) Presence of all IV lines, irrigation solutions and output devices

(C) Fluid balance

(D) All of the above

(36) What are the symptoms of an anaphylactic reaction?

(A) Low blood pressure

(B) Rapid heartbeat

(C) Bronchospasm

(D) All of the above

(37) What is the primary action the surgical team should take in case of an anaphylactic reaction?

(A) Administering antihistamines

(B) Administering epinephrine

(C) Administering steroids

(D) Providing oxygen

(38) What is the primary treatment for malignant hyperthermia?

(A) Obtaining a detailed family history

(B) Monitoring for signs of the disorder during surgery

(C) Administering dantrolene immediately

(D) Decreasing body temperature

(39) What is not part of the approach for treating a surgical site infection?

(A) Wound drainage

(B) Physical therapy

(C) Administration of antibiotics

(D) Oxygen therapy

(40) What is the best treatment for a patient experiencing reactions to anesthesia or difficulty breathing?

(A) Intubation to maintain an open airway

(B) Revision surgery

(C) Administration of blood thinners, such as heparin or warfarin

(D) Wound care

(41) What is the primary treatment for a patient with a hematoma after a surgical procedure?

(A) Physical therapy

(B) Administration of blood thinners, such as heparin or warfarin

(C) Wound care

(D) Topical creams, such as silicone gel or onion extract

(42) A patient who has just undergone surgery is being monitored by a medical-surgical nurse. Which of the following actions should the nurse prioritize in the patient's postoperative care?

(A) Administering pain medication as prescribed by the surgeon

(B) Encouraging the patient to get up and move around as soon as possible

(C) Closely monitoring the patient's condition, vital signs and wound healing and promptly reporting any signs of complications to the surgeon

(D) Allowing the patient to rest without disturbing him for several hours

(43) A patient undergoing a fracture reduction procedure is administered midazolam for moderate sedation. During the procedure, the patient's oxygen saturation levels decrease to below 90% and her heart rate decreases to 40 beats per minute. As a medical-surgical nurse, what would be the most appropriate action to take in this situation?

(A) Administer oxygen through a face mask.

(B) Increase the dose of midazolam.

(C) Notify the surgeon and prepare for intubation.

(D) Wait and observe, as this is a normal reaction to the drug.

(44) Which of the following should be considered when selecting the appropriate level of sedation for a patient according to the ASA Sedation Guidelines?

(A) Type of medication used

(B) Level of sedation achieved

(C) Patient's condition, procedure being performed and patient's preferences

(D) Dosage

(45) What is the significance of conducting a thorough nutritional assessment in medical-surgical patients?

(A) To determine the patient's preferred foods

(B) To improve hospital satisfaction

(C) To prevent malnutrition and its associated health complications

(D) To determine the patient's eating patterns

(46) A BMI value of less than 18.5 indicates which of the following, according to the Food Guide Pyramid guidelines for determining malnutrition?

(A) Healthy weight

(B) Malnutrition

(C) Overweight

(D) Obesity

(47) What is the formula used to calculate BMI if the weight is in pounds and height in inches?

(A) BMI = weight (lb) / height (in)^1

(B) BMI = weight (lb) / height (in)^2

(C) BMI = weight (lb) x 703 / height (in)^2

(D) BMI = weight (lb) / height (in)^2 x 703

(48) A 56-year-old male patient with a history of heart disease and diabetes presents with symptoms of malnutrition, including significant weight loss, fatigue, dry and scaly skin and changes in mental status. Based on the patient's medical history and symptoms, what is the most likely cause of malnutrition in this case?

(A) Inadequate calorie and protein intake

(B) Malabsorption due to gastrointestinal issues

(C) Chronic kidney disease

(D) Increased metabolic demand due to multiple comorbidities

(49) A patient has been assessed, and the following results have been obtained:

- Albumin: 2.5 g/dL (normal range: 3.5–5.5 g/dL)

- Hemoglobin: 10 g/dL (normal range: 13.5–17.5 g/dL)

- Vitamin B12: 80 ng/mL (normal range: 200–1,100 ng/mL)

- C-reactive protein: 8 mg/dL (normal range: 0–5 mg/dL)

Based on these results, what is the most likely diagnosis for this patient?

(A) Vitamin B12 deficiency

(B) Iron deficiency anemia

(C) Malnutrition

(D) Selenium deficiency

(50) What is an indicator of a negative nitrogen balance?

(A) Positive urinary urea nitrogen levels

(B) Increased protein intake

(C) Reduced protein intake

(D) Normal urinary urea nitrogen levels

(51) What is the most common cause of malnutrition among medical-surgical patients?

(A) Malabsorption syndrome

(B) Gastric or bowel resection

(C) Pancreatic insufficiency

(D) Chronic medical conditions

(52) What should be the first step in the process of health care when it comes to patient education?

(A) Develop a teaching plan.

(B) Monitor progress.

(C) Assess the patient's current level of knowledge.

(D) Evaluate the effectiveness of the teaching.

(53) What is the primary focus of the educational process in health care?

(A) To develop a teaching plan

(B) To refer patients to additional resources

(C) To evaluate the effectiveness of the teaching

(D) To empower patients to take an active role in their own health and well-being

(54) What is the purpose of documenting activities and monitoring progress during the implementation of the teaching plan?

(A) To assess the patient's current level of knowledge

(B) To refer the patient to additional resources

(C) To make necessary adjustments in a timely manner

(D) To evaluate the effectiveness of the teaching

(55) Which of the following is an example of evaluating the effectiveness of the teaching plan in the educational process of health care?

(A) Testing skills through return demonstrations

(B) Creating a hypothetical scenario to gauge the patient's response

(C) Allowing the patients to explain their understanding of the topic

(D) All of the above

(56) What is the purpose of documenting the patient's educational process in health care?

(A) To serve as a record of the patient's progress

(B) To provide valuable information for other health care professionals

(C) To make adjustments to the teaching plan as needed

(D) All of the above

(57) Which of the following pieces of information should the nurse document during the educational process in health care?

(A) The patient's learning style

(B) The patient's age and weight

(C) The patient's progress and any adjustments made to the teaching plan

(D) The patient's pain levels

(58) What is the importance of incorporating patient and family input in the educational process in health care?

(A) It increases patient retention and application of information.

(B) It builds a sense of ownership and responsibility for their own learning.

(C) It enhances the use of nursing time.

(D) All of the above.

(59) What are creative methods nurses can use to meet the diverse learning needs of patients and families?

(A) Verbal teaching sessions

(B) Informal teaching methods

(C) Waiting room teaching sessions, printed materials and other multimedia resources

(D) One-on-one teaching sessions

(60) What is the importance of documenting critical information pertaining to patients' conditions before discharge?

(A) It decreases the chances of patients' noncompliance with their health conditions.

(B) It reduces patients' ability to retain and apply the information learned.

(C) It ensures patients have the necessary information and skills to manage their condition and maintain their health after discharge.

(D) It increases the chances of readmission to the health care facility.

(61) A 78-year-old female was admitted to the hospital with chest pain and shortness of breath. She has a history of hypertension and hyperlipidemia. The nurse assigned to the patient was tasked with educating her about her condition, lifestyle modifications and self-care management after discharge. Which of the following is the most important aspect of the educational process for this patient?

(A) Incorporating patient and family input into the educational process

(B) Using waiting-room teaching sessions, printed materials and multimedia resources

(C) Ensuring the patient is aware of critical information before discharge

(D) Building a sense of ownership and responsibility for the patient's learning

(62) What is the definition of health promotion according to the WHO?

(A) The process of improving individual health through health education and instruction

(B) The process of providing community health services

(C) The process of developing care plans to address health risks

(D) The process of advocating for policies and programs that promote health and prevent disease.

(63) Which of the following roles do nurses play in health promotion?

(A) Advocating for policies and programs that promote health

(B) Being the first point of contact for patients and assessing their health risks

(C) Collaborating with other health care professionals and community organizations

(D) All of the above

(64) Which of the following are strategies nurses can employ to improve the overall health of populations?

(A) Primary, secondary and tertiary prevention

(B) Health education and instruction

(C) Collaborating with other health care professionals and community organizations

(D) Assessing patients' health risks and developing care plans

(65) What is the nurse's role in delivering health information and resources to patients?

(A) Providing information and resources to help patients access community health services

(B) Advocating for policies and programs that promote health and prevent disease

(C) Assessing patient's health risks and developing care plans

(D) Collaborating with other health care professionals and community organizations

(66) What is the main focus of tertiary prevention in nursing care?

(A) Reducing the onset of specific diseases

(B) Detecting and treating preclinical pathological changes

(C) Reducing disability or complications and improving patient outcomes

(D) Providing health education and protection

(67) What is the main goal of secondary prevention?

(A) To prevent the onset of specific diseases

(B) To reduce the risk factors for a specific disease

(C) To detect and treat preclinical pathological changes

(D) To reduce the disability or complications arising from a condition

(68) What is an example of tertiary prevention in nursing?

(A) Educating patients on the dangers of smoking

(B) Performing screening procedures for early-stage disease

(C) Providing cardiac rehabilitation following a myocardial infarction

(D) Collaborating with health care professionals to improve the overall health of populations

(69) A nurse encounters a patient who is a heavy smoker. The nurse wants to educate the patient about the dangers of smoking and help him quit the habit. Which of the following types of prevention is the nurse using in this scenario?

(A) Tertiary prevention

(B) Secondary prevention

(C) Primary prevention

(D) No prevention

(70) A nurse encounters a patient who has recently been diagnosed with prediabetic conditions. The nurse wants to detect and treat any early-stage pathological changes to prevent the progression of the disease. Which of the following types of prevention is the nurse using in this scenario?

(A) Tertiary prevention

(B) Secondary prevention

(C) Primary prevention

(D) No prevention

(71) A nurse encounters a patient who has just suffered a myocardial infarction. The nurse wants to reduce the disability and complications arising from the condition and improve the patient's function, longevity and quality of life. Which of the following types of prevention is the nurse using in this scenario?

(A) Tertiary prevention

(B) Secondary prevention

(C) Primary prevention

(D) No prevention

(72) What is a nurse's main role in facilitating access to and use of the health care system?

(A) Making health care more accessible and user-friendly

(B) Providing valuable information and advice about healthy lifestyles

(C) Aiming to empower patients to feel more confident and competent in managing their health

(D) Promoting social change and addressing inequalities

(73) A patient has recently been diagnosed with type 2 diabetes and has many questions about managing the disease. What is the nurse's primary responsibility in this situation?

(A) Facilitating access to and use of the health care system

(B) Promoting health promotion encounters

(C) Providing health information and advice about healthy lifestyles

(D) Promoting social change and addressing inequalities

(74) A patient is feeling overwhelmed and powerless in managing his health. What is the nurse's primary responsibility in this situation?

(A) Health promotion

(B) Providing health information and advice about healthy lifestyles

(C) Empowering the patient

(D) Facilitating access and use of the health care system

(75) A patient is interested in advocating for policies that promote health and prevent disease. What is the nurse's primary responsibility in this situation?

(A) Promoting social change and addressing inequalities

(B) Giving lessons on the different kinds of drugs

(C) Helping the patient become a political activist

(D) Telling the patient that this is too difficult

(76) Which of the following types of resources does a nurse need to be aware of for end-of-life care for a patient and his family?

(A) Home health agencies

(B) Support groups for patients and families

(C) Hospice programs

(D) Financial assistance programs

(77) Which type of resources does a nurse need to be aware of for patients and their families who are struggling to pay for health care costs?

(A) Caregiver support programs

(B) Patient education materials

(C) Financial assistance programs

(D) Advance care planning resources

(78) Which type of resources does a nurse need to be aware of to promote self-management of chronic conditions?

(A) Support groups for patients and families

(B) Patient education materials

(C) Community resources

(D) Referral to specialists

(79) Which type of resources does a nurse need to be aware of for providing respite care for family members?

(A) Community resources

(B) Support groups for patients and families

(C) Caregiver support programs

(D) Patient education materials

(80) What is the importance of evidence-based practice for nurses?

(A) It helps inform their personal opinions.

(B) It helps them make decisions based on the latest research and guidelines.

(C) It helps them make decisions based on the nurse's personal experience.

(D) It helps them make decisions based on patient preferences.

(81) What does a nurse need to be familiar with regarding a patient's medication regimen?

(A) The cost of the medications

(B) The name, dose, frequency and potential side effects of each medication

(C) The manufacturer of the medications

(D) The storage conditions of the medications

(82) What does a nurse need to know about a patient's diagnosis and treatment options?

(A) The cost of the treatments

(B) The patient's insurance coverage

(C) The patient's diagnosis, potential complications and any treatment options that are available

(D) The physician's schedule for follow-up appointments

(83) What is the primary focus of palliative care?

(A) To cure the underlying condition

(B) To extend the patient's life

(C) To manage pain and symptoms and improve quality of life

(D) To perform diagnostic tests to confirm the diagnosis

(84) What is the main goal of palliative care in terms of symptom relief?

(A) To cure the symptoms

(B) To temporarily relieve symptoms

(C) To alleviate symptoms and improve the patient's quality of life

(D) To completely eliminate symptoms

(85) What is the main goal of palliative care in terms of supporting holistic care?

(A) To address only the patient's physical needs

(B) To address the patient's physical, emotional, social and spiritual needs

(C) To address the patient's spiritual needs

(D) To ignore the patient's emotional and social needs

(86) What is the primary focus of palliative care in terms of the dying process?

(A) To extend the patient's life

(B) To hasten death

(C) To provide comfort and support during the dying process

(D) To postpone death

(87) A patient's family is seeking support during their loved one's serious illness. Palliative care can provide _____ to the family.

(A) Physical support

(B) Financial support

(C) Emotional support

(D) Spiritual support

(88) What is the primary goal of hospice care in end-of-life care?

(A) To provide a physical location for care

(B) To cure the patient's illness

(C) To provide comfort and quality of life for individuals nearing the end of their lives

(D) To provide spiritual support

(89) A patient nears the end of her life, and her family is concerned about providing them with spiritual support. Which of the following options would be the most appropriate for the patient and family?

(A) Chaplain services

(B) Traditional healers

(C) Occupational therapy

(D) Online resources

(90) What is the main objective of cultural support in end-of-life care?

(A) To provide access to traditional healers

(B) To offer physical therapy

(C) To provide spiritual counseling

(D) To provide emotional support

(91) Which of the following types of support is often provided as part of end-of-life care?

(A) Traditional healing practices

(B) Religious counseling

(C) Pain management, symptom control and assistance with activities of daily living

(D) Online resources

(92) What is the primary benefit of participating in support groups for patients and caregivers facing end-of-life issues?

(A) Receiving medical treatment and advice

(B) Gaining emotional support and coping mechanisms

(C) Obtaining financial assistance

(D) Finding information about legal matters

(93) What is the purpose of advance directives in end-of-life preferences?

(A) To provide guidance on pain management

(B) To specify a preferred location of care

(C) To outline medical treatment in the event of incapacity

(D) To indicate resuscitation orders

(94) What is the significance of specifying code status in end-of-life preferences?

(A) It provides guidance on pain management.

(B) It determines a preferred location of care.

(C) It outlines medical treatment in the event of incapacity.

(D) It indicates resuscitation orders.

(95) What are some options for end-of-life preferences that can be selected or declined?

(A) Life-sustaining treatments, such as mechanical ventilation or dialysis

(B) Pain management

(C) Family member involvement

(D) Hospice care

(96) Where would an individual prefer to receive care?

(A) At home

(B) In a hospice

(C) In a hospital

(D) Any of the above

(97) What is a living will used for in end-of-life preferences?

(A) Expressing the level of family involvement desired

(B) Specifying medical treatment in case of inability to communicate or make decisions

(C) Determining pain management

(D) Indicating code status

(98) What is the purpose of an advance directive?

(A) To appoint a trusted individual to make health care decisions on behalf of the patient in the event the person becomes incapacitated

(B) To outline an individual's preferences for medical treatment in the event the person becomes incapacitated and unable to communicate

(C) To specify an individual's desire to forgo life-sustaining treatments in the event of a terminal illness or injury

(D) To instruct health care providers to refrain from performing CPR in the event of cardiac or respiratory arrest

(99) What is the purpose of a physician's directive?

(A) To give a lawyer power to make healthcare decisions in case of terminal illness

(B) To give a family member power to make healthcare decisions in case of terminal illness

(C) To specify an individual's desire to forgo life-sustaining treatments in the event of a terminal illness or injury

(D) To instruct health care providers to refrain from performing CPR in the event of cardiac or respiratory arrest

(100) What is the difference between a DNR order and a living will?

(A) A DNR order applies only in the event of cardiac or respiratory arrest, while a living will outlines broader end-of-life preferences.

(B) A DNR order must be signed by a physician to be considered valid, while a living will does not require physician approval.

(C) A DNR order is often requested by the patient's family, while a living will is solely the patient's own decision.

(D) A living will must clearly identify specific treatments the individual wishes to receive or decline, while a DNR order specifies only the refusal of CPR.

(101) What is the purpose of a health care power of attorney?

(A) To outline an individual's end-of-life preferences for medical treatment

(B) To specify an individual's desire to forgo life-sustaining treatments in the event of a terminal illness or injury

(C) To designate a trusted individual to make health care decisions on behalf of the patient in the event the person becomes incapacitated

(D) To instruct health care providers to refrain from performing CPR in the event of cardiac or respiratory arrest

(102) What is a step in the discharge procedure for patients leaving the facility?

(A) Obtaining a written discharge order from the treating physician

(B) Escorting the patient to the exit

(C) Collecting personal belongings from the patient's room

(D) All of the above

(103) What should be included in the written discharge order from the treating physician?

(A) Notifying the patient and the designated family or caregivers of the anticipated discharge date and time.

(B) Any specific instructions for post-discharge care.

(C) Arrangements made with the relevant home care agency or community health facility.

(D) Completed necessary paperwork and consent forms

(104) Which of the following should be done if the patient requires ongoing medical care or assistance upon discharge?

(A) Obtain a written discharge order from the treating physician, including any specific instructions for post-discharge care.

(B) Notify the patient and designated family or caregivers of the anticipated discharge date and time.

(C) If the patient requires ongoing medical care or assistance upon discharge, make sure that appropriate arrangements have been made with the relevant home care agency or community health facility

(D) Ensure that the necessary paperwork and consent forms are complete.

(105) Which of the following is a common symptom of tuberculosis?

(A) Persistent cough lasting three or more weeks

(B) Sudden weight gain

(C) Increased appetite

(D) Skin rash

(106) Which of the following is the most recommended preventative measure for influenza (the flu)?

(A) Wearing gloves at all times

(B) Annual flu vaccination

(C) Taking vitamin C supplements daily

(D) Drinking plenty of water

(107) What is the third step in the discharge procedure?

(A) Write down all facts about the patient

(B) If the patient requires ongoing medical care or assistance upon discharge, make sure that appropriate arrangements have been made with the relevant home care agency or community health facility.

(C) Call the family members of the patient so that they are ready

(D) Check the blood pressure of the patient

(108) What should be reviewed prior to discharge according to the discharge procedure?

(A) The patient's daily routine and lifestyle

(B) The comprehensive medication list for the patient

(C) The patient's individualized discharge care plan

(D) Hands-on demonstration and written instructions for self-care procedures

(109) What should be done to promote medication compliance and prevent improper administration?

(A) Assess the official medication compliance document

(B) Ask the family to be present with the patient

(C) Have a fixed medication schedule that all patients must follow

(D) Align the medication schedule with the patient's daily routine and lifestyle

(110) Which of the following should be provided for self-care procedures or treatments that the patient or the family will perform at home?

(A) Review of any self-care procedures or treatments that the patient or the family will need to perform at home.

(B) Hands-on demonstration and written instructions

(C) A comprehensive medication list for the patient

(D) Follow up to ensure that the patient and the family understand the procedures and are able to perform them correctly

(111) Which group is considered high-risk and is strongly advised to get the annual flu vaccination?

(A) Healthy adults with no underlying conditions

(B) Teenagers who participate in sports activities

(C) Pregnant women and individuals with chronic illnesses

(D) People who live in tropical climates

(112) What is the fifth step in the discharge procedure?

(A) Create a comprehensive medication list for the patient.

(B) Review and discuss the patient's individualized discharge care plan with the patient and the family or designated caregivers.

(C) Review any self-care procedures or treatments that the patient or the family will need to perform at home.

(D) Obtain a written discharge order from the treating physician, including any specific instructions for post-discharge care.

(113) Mr. Arkin was admitted to the hospital for a heart condition. What is the most important step taken during the discharge process to ensure his smooth transition back home?

(A) Notifying Mr. Arkin and his family of the anticipated discharge date and time

(B) Obtaining a written discharge order from the treating physician

(C) Reviewing and discussing Mr. Arkin's individualized discharge care plan with him and his family

(D) Creating a comprehensive medication list for Mr. Arkin

(114) Mrs. Lewis required ongoing medical care after her hospital discharge. Which of the following was the most critical step taken in the discharge procedure to ensure her continued care at home?

(A) Notifying Mrs. Lewis and her family of the anticipated discharge date and time

(B) Obtaining a written discharge order from the treating physician

(C) Making sure appropriate arrangements have been made with the relevant home care agency or community health facility

(D) Reviewing any self-care procedures or treatments that Mrs. Lewis and her family will need to perform at home

(115) What was the most critical step taken to confirm Mr. Olivares's follow-up appointment after his discharge?

(A) Retrieving personal belongings

(B) Providing dietary instructions

(C) Confirming a follow-up appointment with the physician

(D) Obtaining signature on receipt of valuables

(116) When preparing for Mr. Jackson's discharge from the hospital, what is the most important step?

(A) Obtaining a written discharge order from the treating physician

(B) Reviewing self-care procedures with the patient and his family

(C) Confirming follow-up appointment with the physician

(D) Retrieving personal belongings and obtaining a signature on receipt of valuables

(117) What is the first step a nurse should take when a patient is ready to leave the facility?

(A) Collect the patient's personal belongings.

(B) Conduct a final check of the patient's room.

(C) Help the patient into a wheelchair or onto a stretcher.

(D) Strip the bed linens.

(118) What is patient- and family-centered care, and what is the aim of this approach?

(A) Patient- and family-centered care is a traditional approach to health care that emphasizes collaboration between health care providers and patients.

(B) Patient- and family-centered care is a person-centered approach to health care that values the unique needs and perspectives of patients and their families and emphasizes collaboration and partnership between health care providers, patients and families.

(C) Patient- and family-centered care is a medical approach to health care that addresses only the physical needs of patients.

(D) Patient- and family-centered care is an approach to health care that addresses only the emotional and psychological needs of patients and their families.

(119) What is the primary focus of the respect and dignity principle in patient- and family-centered care?

(A) Providing clear and complete information

(B) Encouraging active patient and family participation

(C) Valuing the unique needs and perspectives of patients and families

(D) Collaborating with health care practitioners

(120) What is the goal of collaboration in patient- and family-centered care?

(A) To provide patients and families with clear information

(B) To empower patients and families to take an active role in their care

(C) To promote teamwork and cooperation between all stakeholders in health care

(D) To support patients and families in making informed decisions about their treatment

(121) What is the main goal of care coordination in health care?

(A) To ensure that the patient's needs are met throughout the care process

(B) To facilitate the movement of patients from one level of care to another

(C) To implement automated workflows and real-time transition data

(D) To provide clear communication between providers and staff

(122) What is the main benefit of implementing automated workflows in the care coordination process?

(A) Improving the efficiency and accuracy of the process

(B) Providing real-time transition data

(C) Enhancing communication across providers and staff

(D) Promoting proper planning

(123) What is the main focus of interprofessional roles and responsibilities in health care?

(A) The division of tasks among health care professionals

(B) Individualized patient care

(C) Diagnosis and treatment planning

(D) Patient education and ongoing care coordination

(124) What is the main focus of physical therapists and occupational therapists working together in patient care?

(A) Diagnosis and treatment planning

(B) Improving physical strength and mobility

(C) Regaining the ability to perform daily activities

(D) Connecting patients with community resources

(125) What is the role of a pharmacist in collaborating with physicians to ensure patient care?

(A) Administering medication

(B) Reviewing medication history and making recommendations to the physician

(C) Making the final decision on appropriate medication

(D) Monitoring vital signs

(126) Who is responsible for coordinating care for patients with complex needs in an interdisciplinary team of health care professionals?

(A) Physician

(B) Nurse

(C) Social worker

(D) Case manager

(127) What is the main focus of physical therapy in an interprofessional health care team?

(A) Improving physical strength and mobility

(B) Helping patients recover from injuries or illnesses

(C) Administering medication

(D) Connecting patients with community resources

(128) What is the primary purpose of a surgical retractor?

(A) To cut through tissue during a surgical procedure

(B) To control bleeding by clamping off blood vessels

(C) To hold back underlying organs or tissues, providing access to the surgical site

(D) To suture and close surgical incisions

(129) A surgeon requests a scalpel during a procedure. What is the main function of this tool?

(A) To suture and close the surgical wound

(B) To dilate body openings for improved visibility

(C) To cut or dissect tissue during surgery

(D) To clamp blood vessels and control bleeding

(130) What is the first level of care within a continuum of care?

(A) Acute care

(B) Prevention and wellness

(C) Primary care

(D) End-of-life care

(131) Which of the following types of care is provided by a patient's primary care physician or nurse practitioner?

(A) Acute care

(B) End-of-life care

(C) Primary care

(D) Rehabilitation

(132) Which of the following types of care is focused on helping patients recover from illness or injury?

(A) Acute care

(B) End-of-life care

(C) Primary care

(D) Rehabilitation

(133) Which of the following types of care is focused on comfort and support for patients nearing the end of life?

(A) Acute care

(B) End-of-life care

(C) Primary care

(D) Rehabilitation

(134) Which of the following types of care is provided for patients with chronic conditions that require ongoing management and support?

(A) Prevention and wellness

(B) Primary care

(C) Acute care

(D) Long-term care

(135) What is the main role of medical-surgical nurses in the preoperative phase of surgery?

(A) To educate the patient about the procedure

(B) To assess the patient's medical history

(C) To ensure patient preparation for the procedure

(D) All of the above

(136) Medical-surgical nurses _____ in the postoperative phase of surgery.

(A) Work with the surgical team

(B) Review the patient's medical history

(C) Provide care to the patient

(D) None of the above

(137) Medical-surgical nurses are responsible for _____ during surgery.

(A) Monitoring the patient's vital signs

(B) Providing support to the surgical team

(C) Administering medication

(D) All of the above.

(138) A medical-surgical nurse is caring for a patient who has just undergone surgery. Which of the following should the nurse prioritize in the care plan for this patient?

(A) Monitoring the patient's vital signs

(B) Managing pain

(C) Providing education to the patient and family

(D) Collaborating with the health care team

(139) What are the common factors that increase a patient's risk for readmission to the hospital?

(A) Chronic conditions, such as heart failure, COPD and diabetes

(B) Recent surgical procedure or discharge from the ICU

(C) Poor communication between health care providers

(D) All of the above

(140) What are the three categories in the Donabedian model for evaluating the quality of health care organizations?

(A) Outcome, progress and structure

(B) Structure, outcome and process

(C) Process, structure and efficiency

(D) Quality, cost and efficiency

(141) What is an example of a structural measure in the health care industry?

(A) The utilization of EHRs

(B) The proportion of board-certified physicians

(C) The ratio of providers to patients

(D) All of the above

(142) What is an example of a process measure used to assess the quality of care provided by a health care provider?

(A) The overall space inside of the hospital

(B) The total number of pharmacists, nurses and physicians

(C) Proportion of patients who receive preventive services

(D) The operating hours of the hospital

(143) What is the purpose of outcome measures in evaluating health care quality?

(A) To evaluate the utilization of systems and processes put in place by health care providers

(B) To assess the steps taken by health care providers to ensure and improve patient health

(C) To evaluate the impact of health care services or interventions on the health status of patients

(D) To highlight the extent to which health care providers emphasize promoting health and avoiding illnesses

(144) Antiviral drugs for treating the flu are most effective when taken _____.

(A) Before the flu season starts

(B) At any time during the illness

(C) Within the first 48 hours after symptoms start

(D) After the flu symptoms have subsided

(145) What is the purpose of documenting nurses' work?

(A) To communicate effectively with other members of the health care team

(B) To provide information for professionals involved in accreditation, credentialing, legal, regulatory, reimbursement, research and quality activities

(C) To ensure continuity of care

(D) All of the above

(146) What are the characteristics of high-quality nursing documentation?

(A) Inaccurate and inconsistent

(B) Accessible, accurate and relevant

(C) Unclear and incomplete

(D) Timeless and not retrievable

(147) Which of the following attributes is most important for high-quality nursing documentation?

(A) Timeliness

(B) Clarity

(C) Auditability

(D) Relevance

(148) Which of the following best describes the purpose of EHRs?

(A) To store patient demographic information

(B) To reduce medical errors and improve patient care

(C) To increase the cost-effectiveness of health care

(D) To facilitate the sharing of information between health care providers

(149) What is a key component of downtime procedures in health care organizations?

(A) Establishing communication protocols

(B) Ignoring critical patient populations

(C) Failing to document incidents

(D) Not training staff

(150) What is a downtime procedure in health care?

(A) A way to manage patients who are in critical condition during an emergency

(B) A process to ensure the availability of medical supplies during a shortage

(C) A procedure to handle system outages and disruptions to minimize the impact on patient care

(D) A plan to manage patient flow in the event of a disaster

Test 2: Answers & Explanations

(1) (B) The use of multiple medications.

This can happen when a patient takes multiple medications to treat the same condition or when a medication does not match the diagnosis. It can also occur when a patient takes several medications that have similar actions to treat multiple conditions simultaneously or mixes nutritional supplements or herbal products with medications.

(2) (D) All of the above.

Older adults may take over-the-counter (OTC) preparations to alleviate symptoms such as pain, constipation, insomnia and indigestion. Children and patients with mental illnesses may also be at risk due to the use of multiple medications to treat different conditions.

(3) (C) Regularly review the patient's medication list and adjust or reduce the number of medications as necessary.

To minimize the risks associated with polypharmacy in this case, the health care provider should regularly review the patient's medication list and make adjustments as necessary. This could involve reducing the number of medications or changing the dosage to prevent adverse reactions and medication interactions.

(4) (A) To identify potential issues in a patient's medication list.

This helps health care providers ensure that patients are receiving the right medications for their specific needs.

(5) (B) Contamination of the water supply and harm to wildlife.

When medications are flushed down the toilet or thrown in the trash, they can enter the water supply and harm aquatic life. Improper disposal of medication also poses a risk to human health if not handled properly. It is important to follow the proper disposal instructions or take them to a medication take-back program or designated disposal site.

(6) (A) Assessing pain.

This allows health care providers to understand the severity, location and nature of a patient's pain and identify any underlying causes. Assessing pain can be done through various tools and methods, including subjective pain assessment tools, visual aids, questionnaires and observing for objective signs.

(7) (A) As either acute or chronic.

Acute pain is mild to severe pain that has a rapid onset and lasts less than six months, while chronic pain lasts beyond the expected healing time and may be challenging to relate to the original injury or tissue damage. This classification helps health care providers understand the nature and duration of a patient's pain and develop an appropriate treatment plan.

(8) (D) Develop a pain management plan that includes a combination of medication and nonmedication options.

The 0–10 rating scale is a subjective tool that helps determine the severity of pain. A score of 8 indicates that the patient is experiencing severe pain and the health care provider should develop a comprehensive pain management plan that includes a combination of medication and nonmedication options, such as physical therapy, occupational therapy, counseling or relaxation techniques.

(9) (B) Nonsteroidal anti-inflammatory drugs (NSAIDs), acetaminophen and opioid analgesics.

These medications can be administered in different ways, such as orally, parenterally, intraspinal and topically. Nurses may also assist with the administration of regional anesthesia techniques, such as epidurals, spinal blocks and nerve blocks, as well as with patient-controlled analgesia (PCA) systems and scheduled dosing regimens.

(10) (D) Physical therapy, cognitive-behavioral therapy and occupational therapy.

These treatments be accompanied by medications, such as antidepressants, anticonvulsants and muscle relaxants and with the administration of TENS and spinal cord stimulation. These nonpharmacologic interventions focus on helping patients manage their pain and improve their overall quality of life.

(11) Answer: (A) 1-4 days

The incubation period refers to the time from when a person is first exposed to the flu virus and infected, to when symptoms begin. For the flu, this is typically about 1-4 days, with an average of about 2 days. This means that you could pass the flu to someone else before you even know you're sick, as well as while you're sick. This is why flu prevention measures like vaccination, good hygiene practices, and staying away from others while ill are so important.

(12) (B) Advise the patient to continue taking the medication as prescribed and inform the physician of the lack of improvement.

Chronic pain management may require a combination of medication, nonpharmacologic interventions and close monitoring. Increasing the dosage of the medication without consulting the physician, stopping the medication without consulting the physician or suggesting alternative pain management methods without consulting the physician may put the patient at risk.

(13) (D) All of the above.

This approach can include a combination of pharmacological and nonpharmacologic interventions to target different aspects of the pain experience. The benefits of a multimodal approach include the ability to target multiple pain pathways, reduce the risk of side effects and improve pain control.

(14) (C) Assess the patient's pain using a validated pain assessment tool, document the results and administer medication per the physician's order.

This is the protocol the nurse should follow to ensure that the patient's pain is effectively managed and that the individual receives appropriate care.

(15) (B) Respect the patient's discomfort and suggest alternative methods for communicating about her pain.

Patient advocacy in pain management includes listening to patients' concerns and understanding their pain experience. The nurse should respect the patient's discomfort and suggest alternative methods for communicating about pain.

(16) (C) Discuss the patient's cultural beliefs with the interdisciplinary team and work to develop a culturally sensitive treatment plan.

Patient advocacy in pain management includes being aware of any cultural, linguistic or physical barriers to effective pain management. Ignoring patients' cultural beliefs, informing patients that their cultural beliefs are incorrect or advising the patients to ignore their cultural beliefs and follow the treatment plan are not appropriate actions.

(17) (C) Consult with other members of the health care team, including pain specialists and physical therapists, to determine the most appropriate nonpharmacological pain management method.

Collaborating with other members of the health care team to provide comprehensive pain management, including consulting with pain specialists, physical therapists and other specialists as needed, is an important aspect of nonpharmacological pain management.

(18) (B) To stimulate the skin and underlying tissues to alleviate pain and improve circulation.

Techniques such as heat therapy and cold therapy are used to stimulate the skin and underlying tissues, providing temporary relief from pain and discomfort.

(19) (C) By inserting needles into special points on the body to balance the flow of energy and alleviate pain.

These points correspond to different pathways or channels in the body called meridians, which are believed to be connected to the flow of energy throughout the body. Stimulating these acupoints aims to balance the flow of energy and alleviate pain.

(20) (D) Using techniques such as relaxation, visualization and mindfulness to manage pain.

Cognitive and behavioral pain management is an approach that focuses on using techniques such as relaxation, visualization and mindfulness to manage pain rather than solely relying on medication.

(21) (D) By enabling an individual to control certain physiological processes to manage pain and other symptoms.

This technique typically involves the use of electronic sensors and monitoring equipment to provide patients with feedback on their physiological state.

(22) (D) By using essential oils from plants to promote physical and psychological well-being by stimulating the olfactory system and activating certain areas of the brain.

Aromatherapy is a form of CAM that uses essential oils from plants to promote physical and psychological well-being.

(23) (A) To document the patient's understanding and agreement to the procedure.

Obtaining informed consent from the patient prior to the procedure is an important step in ensuring that the patient understands the procedure, its risks and benefits and any alternative options. The patient's signature on a consent form serves as documentation of the person's understanding and agreement to the procedure.

(24) (B) To ensure the correct patient, procedure and site are being worked on.

A time-out is a pause in the surgical procedure when the surgical team will verbally confirm the patient's identity, the procedure to be performed and the surgical site before proceeding with the surgery. This is an important step in ensuring patient safety.

(25) (C) To monitor patients' well-being and ensure that they are stable.

Monitoring the patient's vital signs before, during and after the procedure is important to ensure the patient's well-being and identify any potential complications early. This includes monitoring the patient's heart rate, blood pressure, oxygen saturation and temperature, as well as any other vital signs that are relevant to the specific procedure.

(26) (C) To prevent postoperative infection.

Cefazolin (Ancef) is an antibiotic medication that is used to prevent postoperative infection in patients. It works by stopping the growth of bacteria, which can cause infection.

(27) (D) To reduce acid secretion and gastric volume.

Famotidine (Pepcid) is a histamine H2-receptor antagonist medication that works by reducing acid secretion and gastric volume in the stomach. This medication is used to treat conditions such as acid reflux and gastritis.

(28) (C) To reduce oral and respiratory secretions.

Atropine (Isopto Atropine) is an anticholinergic medication that works by blocking the action of a neurotransmitter called acetylcholine. This results in the reduction of oral and respiratory secretions, which can be useful in certain medical procedures, such as bronchoscopy or intubation.

(29) (C) To induce sedation, anxiety and amnesic effects.

Midazolam (Versed) is a sedative medication that works by slowing down the activity of the central nervous system. This results in sedation, anxiety relief and amnesic effects. It is often used before procedures, such as endoscopy or dental surgery, to help patients relax and reduce anxiety.

(30) (D) All of the above.

The PACU is a critical part of the recovery process for patients after surgery. The PACU is specifically designed to provide close monitoring and care during this period, minimizing the need for transportation and ensuring that patients receive the care they need in a timely manner. It is located adjacent to the OR, and the level of care provided in the PACU is tailored to the patient's individual needs and divided into three phases.

(31) (D) Implementing a combination of pharmacological and nonpharmacological pain management methods.

The most appropriate method of pain management for a patient in the PACU will depend on the patient's individual needs and condition. The patient's medical history, current medications and current vital signs should be considered when determining the most appropriate pain management method.

(32) (C) Assessing the patient's ABC status.

The first step in post-surgery patient care is to ensure that the patient's airway, breathing and circulation are stable and that any signs of inadequate oxygenation and ventilation are identified and treated promptly.

(33) (B) Pulse oximetry.

Pulse oximetry is a noninvasive means of measuring oxygen levels in the blood and can provide valuable information about the patient's oxygenation status after surgery.

(34) (A) Residual sensory or motor blockade.

In patients who have received a regional anesthetic, it is important to check for any residual sensory or motor blockade, as this can affect the patient's mobility and ability to perform activities of daily living. It is also important to explain all activities to the patient from the moment of admission to the PACU.

(35) (D) All of the above.

When assessing a patient's urinary system after surgery, it is important to note the input and output measurements, the presence of all IV lines, irrigation solutions and output devices, such as catheters and wound drains, as well as evaluating fluid balance. It is important to monitor these aspects of the patient's urinary system to ensure that the patient is receiving the appropriate amount of fluid and that any output devices are functioning properly.

(36) (D) All of the above.

The symptoms of an anaphylactic reaction include low blood pressure, rapid heartbeat, bronchospasm and possible fluid accumulation in the lungs. It is crucial for the surgical team to be aware of these symptoms and act quickly to mitigate potential harm to the patient.

(37) (B) Administering epinephrine.

In case of an anaphylactic reaction, the primary action that should be taken is administering epinephrine. This medication is essential to stop the progression of the allergic reaction and save the patient's life.

(38) (C) Administering dantrolene immediately.

It is critical for medical professionals to be aware of the possibility of malignant hyperthermia and take appropriate precautions, such as obtaining a detailed family history and monitoring for signs of the disorder during surgery.

(39) (D) Oxygen therapy.

The approach for treating a surgical site infection includes wound drainage, administration of antibiotics and reopening of the surgical site if necessary. A wound vacuum or vacuum-assisted closure device may also be used to remove infected material and promote healing.

(40) (A) Intubation to maintain an open airway.

The best treatment for a patient experiencing reactions to anesthesia or difficulty breathing may include oxygen therapy, medication, and in severe cases, intubation to maintain an open airway.

(41) (B) Administration of blood thinners, such as heparin or warfarin.

The treatment for a patient with a hematoma after a surgical procedure also involves drainage of the affected area using a needle and syringe or a small incision. In some cases, a pressure dressing may be applied to reduce swelling.

(42) (C) Closely monitoring the patient's condition, vital signs and wound healing and promptly reporting any signs of complications to the surgeon.

Medical-surgical nurses should closely monitor the patient's condition, vital signs and wound healing and promptly report and document any signs of complications to the surgeon. Nursing care should be individualized based on the patient's needs and the surgeon's postoperative instructions.

(43) (C) Notify the surgeon and prepare for intubation.

If the patient's oxygen saturation levels decrease to below 90% and the heart rate decreases to 40 beats per minute, it is indicative of a potential airway obstruction or cardiac event. As a medical-surgical nurse, it is crucial to immediately notify the surgeon and prepare for intubation to ensure the patient's safety and well-being.

(44) (C) Patient's condition, procedure being performed and patient's preferences.

The ASA Sedation Guidelines protocol states that the appropriate level of sedation should be selected based on the patient's condition, the procedure being performed and the patient's preferences.

(45) (C) To prevent malnutrition and its associated health complications.

A well-rounded and balanced diet is essential for the body to function properly and prevent malnutrition, which can lead to significant health complications. By conducting a thorough nutritional assessment, health care providers can identify any deficiencies or imbalances in the patient's diet and take appropriate steps to prevent malnutrition.

(46) (B) Malnutrition.

A BMI value of less than 18.5 is considered malnutrition, according to the Food Guide Pyramid guidelines, as it indicates that the patient is underweight.

(47) (D) BMI = weight (lb) / height (in)^2 x 703.

The formula for calculating BMI when the weight is in pounds and height is in inches is BMI = weight (lb) / height (in)^2 x 703.

(48) (D) Increased metabolic demand due to multiple comorbidities.

The patient has a history of heart disease and diabetes, which both increase the body's metabolic demand and can lead to malnutrition if not properly managed. Additionally, the patient's symptoms, including weight loss and fatigue, suggest that the body is not getting the nutrients it needs to function properly.

(49) (C) Malnutrition.

The patient's low albumin level (2.5 g/dL) and elevated CRP level (8 mg/dL) are consistent with malnutrition. Additionally, the low hemoglobin level (10 g/dL) and low vitamin B12 level (80 ng/mL) can be complications of malnutrition, leading to anemia. Therefore, the most likely diagnosis for this patient is malnutrition.

(50) (C) Reduced protein intake.

A negative nitrogen balance occurs when the losses of nitrogen exceed the intake, which is an indication of protein deficiency. This can be seen in conditions such as malnutrition, chronic illness and injury and is indicated by a reduced protein intake.

(51) (D) Chronic medical conditions.

Chronic medical conditions, such as cancer, heart failure, kidney disease and diabetes, are the most common cause of malnutrition among medical-surgical patients. These conditions increase the risk of malnutrition due to increased energy and nutrient requirements, decreased appetite and increased metabolic rate.

(52) (C) Assess the patient's current level of knowledge.

The first step when it comes to patient education is to assess the patient's current level of knowledge. This information is used to develop a teaching plan that outlines clear learning objectives, relevant content and effective teaching methods.

(53) (D) To empower patients to take an active role in their own health and well-being.

The primary focus of the educational process in health care is to empower the patients to take an active role in their own health and well-being. The process begins with assessing patients' current level of knowledge and is followed by the development of a teaching plan that outlines clear learning objectives and relevant content.

(54) (C) To make necessary adjustments in a timely manner.

The purpose of documenting activities and monitoring progress during the implementation of the teaching plan is to ensure that any necessary adjustments are made in a timely manner. The health care professional must continuously assess and evaluate the patient's understanding and progress in order to adapt their teaching strategies as needed.

(55) (D) All of the above.

An example of evaluating the effectiveness of teaching in the educational process of health care is testing skills through return demonstrations, creating a hypothetical scenario to gauge the patient's response and allowing the patient to explain their understanding of the topic. These methods allow the health care professional to gauge the patient's understanding and progress, ensuring that the educational experience is personalized and effective.

(56) (D) All of the above.

Documentation is an essential aspect of the educational process in health care and serves as a record of the patient's progress, provides valuable information for other health care professionals and can be used to make adjustments to the teaching plan as needed.

(57) (C) The patient's progress and any adjustments made to the teaching plan.

The nurse is responsible for documenting the patient's progress and any adjustments made to the teaching plan during the educational process. This documentation not only serves as a record of the patient's progress but also provides valuable information for other health care professionals involved in the patient's care. The nurse should also document the data used to assess the patient and the actions taken as a result of the assessment.

(58) (D) All of the above.

Incorporating patient and family input into the educational process is important for achieving long-term success, as it increases patient retention and application of information, builds a sense of ownership and responsibility for their own learning and enhances the use of nursing time.

(59) (C) Waiting-room teaching sessions, printed materials and other multimedia resources.

Nurses can use creative methods, such as waiting room teaching sessions, printed materials and other multimedia resources, to meet the diverse learning needs of patients and families. These methods allow nurses to provide targeted and relevant education in a variety of settings, increasing the chances that the patient will retain and apply the information learned.

(60) (C) It ensures patients have the necessary information and skills to manage their condition and maintain their health after discharge.

This is an important aspect of the educational process as it ensures patients have the necessary information and skills to manage their condition and maintain their health after discharge.

(61) (C) Ensuring the patient is aware of critical information before discharge.

This is an important aspect of the educational process, as it ensures the patient has the necessary information and skills to manage their condition and maintain their health after discharge.

(62) (A) The process of improving individual health through health education and instruction.

The WHO defines health promotion as the process of giving individuals the tools and resources to improve their health and increase control over it.

(63) (D) All of the above.

Nurses have a pivotal role in health promotion and are responsible for a variety of tasks to improve the health and well-being of individuals, families and communities. As experienced and educated health care professionals, they are the first point of contact for patients, assess patients' health risks, provide information and resources, advocate for policies and programs and collaborate with other health care professionals and community organizations.

(64) (A) Primary, secondary and tertiary prevention.

Nurses can employ various strategies to improve the overall health of populations. One of these strategies is the use of primary, secondary and tertiary prevention. These strategies allow nurses to address health risks, prevent disease and promote overall health and well-being.

(65) (A) Providing information and resources to help patients access community health services.

Nurses are often the first point of contact for patients and are responsible for delivering accurate and pertinent health information through health education and instruction. They also provide information and resources to help patients access community health services.

(66) (C) Reducing disability or complications and improving patient outcomes.

This type of prevention aims to improve a patient's function, longevity and quality of life by reducing the impact of a condition through interventions and treatments that focus on restoring the patient's physical and emotional health.

(67) (C) To detect and treat pre-clinical pathological changes.

Secondary prevention is focused on detecting and treating pre-clinical pathological changes, which are the changes that occur before a disease becomes apparent. This type of prevention aims to control the progression of the disease so that patients can receive treatment early and prevent it from becoming more serious.

(68) (C) Providing cardiac rehabilitation following a myocardial infarction.

Tertiary prevention aims to reduce the disability or complications arising from a condition and improve a patient's function, longevity and quality of life. In this type of prevention, nurses may provide rehabilitation services to help patients recover from a heart attack. For example, cardiac rehabilitation may involve encouraging patients to make lifestyle changes, such as losing weight, to reduce the likelihood of a recurrence.

(69) (C) Primary prevention.

The nurse is attempting to prevent the onset of a disease (in this case, respiratory disease) by reducing a risk factor (smoking) through education and protection. This is an example of primary prevention.

(70) (B) Secondary prevention.

The nurse is attempting to detect and treat pre-clinical pathological changes to control the progression of the disease (in this case, diabetes).

(71) (A) Tertiary prevention.

The nurse is attempting to reduce the disability and complications arising from a condition (in this case, a myocardial infarction) and improve the patient's function, longevity and quality of life.

(72) (A) Making health care more accessible and user-friendly.

Nurses make health care more accessible and user-friendly by helping patients navigate the health care system and understand their health care options.

(73) (C) Providing health information and advice about healthy lifestyles.

In this case, the nurse's primary responsibility is to provide the patient with information and advice about managing their type 2 diabetes and adopting a healthy lifestyle to manage the disease effectively. The nurse can provide the patient with information about diet, physical activity and self-management techniques.

(74) (C) Empowering the patient.

In this case, the nurse's primary responsibility is to empower patients to feel more confident and competent in managing their health. The nurse can help patients develop personal skills and strategies to take control of their health and improve their overall well-being.

(75) (A) Promoting social change and addressing inequalities.

In this case, the nurse's primary responsibility is to promote social change and address inequalities by advocating for policies and programs that promote health and prevent disease. The nurse can collaborate with other health care professionals and community organizations to improve the overall health of populations and help patients access community health services.

(76) (C) Hospice programs.

A nurse needs to be aware of a local hospice program, as it provides care and support for patients and their families during the end-of-life process. Services may include symptom management, emotional and spiritual support and respite care for family members. The nurse needs to know how to refer patients and families to the hospice program and work with the hospice team to provide coordinated care.

(77) (C) Financial assistance programs.

A nurse needs to be aware of financial assistance programs for patients and families who may be struggling to pay for health care costs. These programs can help patients and their families with the cost of health care, making it more accessible and manageable.

(78) (B) Patient education materials.

A nurse needs to be aware of patient education materials and information on self-management of chronic conditions. These materials can provide valuable information and guidance to patients to help them manage their conditions effectively.

(79) (C) Caregiver support programs.

A nurse needs to be aware of caregiver support programs and respite care services. These programs and services provide support to family members who are caring for a loved one, including respite care to give them a break from caregiving responsibilities.

(80) (B) It helps them make decisions based on the latest research and guidelines.

Evidence-based practice is a crucial aspect of nursing and involves using the latest research and guidelines to inform clinical decision-making and patient care. By using evidence-based practice, nurses can ensure that their practice is based on the most current and accurate information available and that they are providing the best possible care to their patients.

(81) (B) The name, dose, frequency and potential side effects of each medication.

Nurses need to be familiar with the patient's medication regimen, including important details such as the name, dose, frequency and potential side effects of each medication. This information is critical in ensuring that the patient receives safe and effective care.

(82) (C) The patient's diagnosis, potential complications and any treatment options that are available.

A nurse needs to know the patient's diagnosis, potential complications and any treatment options that are available. This information is crucial for providing effective and appropriate care to patients. By being knowledgeable about the patient's condition and treatment options, a nurse can provide accurate information to the patient and the family and help promote patient satisfaction.

(83) (C) To manage pain and symptoms and improve quality of life.

The primary focus of palliative care is to manage pain and symptoms and improve the quality of life for patients living with serious, advanced or terminal illnesses. It does not focus on trying to cure the underlying condition, but rather aims to alleviate symptoms and make the patient more comfortable.

(84) (C) To alleviate symptoms and improve the patient's quality of life.

The main goal of palliative care in terms of symptom relief is to alleviate symptoms such as pain, nausea and fatigue and improve the patient's quality of life. This type of care recognizes the importance of managing symptoms and reducing suffering and seeks to provide patients with the necessary treatments and support to achieve this goal.

(85) (B) To address the patient's physical, emotional, social and spiritual needs.

This type of care recognizes the importance of a comprehensive approach to care and seeks to enhance the patient's quality of life by addressing all aspects of their well-being. This may include managing symptoms, providing emotional and spiritual support, addressing social needs and helping the patient maintain independence and dignity.

(86) (C) To provide comfort and support during the dying process.

The primary focus of palliative care in terms of the dying process is to provide comfort and support. Palliative care recognizes that dying is a normal part of life and seeks to make the process as comfortable and dignified as possible for the patient and their family. This may involve managing symptoms, providing emotional and spiritual support and addressing other needs.

(87) (C) Emotional support.

In the case of a patient's family seeking support during their loved one's serious illness, palliative care can provide emotional support through counseling and grief support. This helps the family cope with the stress and loss associated with their loved one's condition and provides a safe and supportive space for them to process their emotions.

(88) (C) To provide comfort and quality of life for individuals nearing the end of their lives.

Hospice care is not just a physical location but rather a concept of care that prioritizes compassion, concern and support for individuals who are nearing the end of their lives. Its main goal is to provide comfort and quality of life by focusing on symptom management, advance care planning, spiritual support and family assistance rather than trying to cure the patient's illness.

(89) (A) Chaplain services.

Those services provide spiritual counseling and support to individuals and their families during the end-of-life process. They can offer comfort, guidance and support in a patient's spiritual or religious beliefs, helping ease the emotional stress that can often accompany this stage of life.

(90) (A) To provide access to traditional healers.

Cultural support in end-of-life care aims to take into account the individual's cultural background and provide access to traditional healers or cultural practices that may provide comfort and support. This may include respecting dietary restrictions or other cultural needs that are important to the individual.

(91) (C) Pain management, symptom control and assistance with activities of daily living.

Physical support is an important aspect of end-of-life care and can include pain management, symptom control and assistance with activities of daily living. This can be done through the provision of medication, as well as nonmedical interventions, such as occupational, physical or speech therapy.

(92) (B) Gaining emotional support and coping mechanisms.

Gaining emotional support and coping mechanisms is the primary benefit of participating in support groups for patients and caregivers facing end-of-life issues. According to the information provided, support groups provide emotional support and help people cope with end-of-life issues.

(93) (C) To outline medical treatment in the event of incapacity.

To outline medical treatment in the event of incapacity is the purpose of advance directives in end-of-life preferences. Advance directives are used to outline their preferences for medical treatment, such as a living will, in case they become unable to communicate or make decisions for themselves.

(94) (D) It indicates resuscitation orders.

End-of-life preferences encompass decisions about important medical matters and care, including specifying whether an individual would like to receive cardiopulmonary resuscitation in the event of cardiac or respiratory arrest. This is known as code status or DNR orders.

(95) (A) Life-sustaining treatments, such as mechanical ventilation or dialysis.

One of the options for end-of-life preferences is the selection or decline of certain life-sustaining treatments, such as mechanical ventilation or dialysis.

(96) (D) Any of the above.

An individual's preferences for the location of their end-of-life care can vary. Some may prefer to receive care at home, where they feel comfortable and surrounded by loved ones. Others may prefer a hospice or hospital setting for access to medical resources and support. The decision of where to receive care is an important aspect of end-of-life preferences.

(97) (B) Specifying medical treatment in case of inability to communicate or make decisions.

A living will is a type of advance directive that outlines an individual's preferences for medical treatment in the event that they become unable to communicate or make decisions for themselves. This document helps ensure that their end-of-life wishes are honored and respected even if they are unable to express them directly.

(98) (B) To outline an individual's preferences for medical treatment in the event the person becomes incapacitated and unable to communicate.

An advance directive is a legally binding document that allows an individual to specify their preferences for medical treatment in the event the person becomes incapacitated and unable to communicate. It must comply with state-specific guidelines and regulations.

(99) (C) To specify an individual's desire to forgo life-sustaining treatments in the event of a terminal illness or injury.

A physician's directive is a written statement that outlines an individual's desire to forgo life-sustaining treatments in the event of a terminal illness or injury. It indicates specific measures to be used or withheld.

(100) (A) A DNR order applies only in the event of cardiac or respiratory arrest, while a living will outlines broader end-of-life preferences.

A DNR order is often requested by the patient's family and must be signed by a physician to be considered valid. On the other hand, a living will is a document that outlines an individual's preferences for medical treatment and end-of-life care in the event the person becomes incapacitated and unable to communicate.

(101) (C) To designate a trusted individual to make health care decisions on behalf of the patient in the event they become incapacitated.

This document grants a designated individual the legal authority to make decisions about the patient's health care in the event the individual is unable to do so for him or herself. It does not outline end-of-life preferences for medical treatment, specify a desire to forgo life-sustaining treatments or instruct health care providers on specific measures to be used or withheld.

(102) (D) All of the above.

Obtaining a written discharge order from the treating physician is step 2 in the discharge procedure. Escorting the patient to the exit is step 14 in the procedure.

Collecting personal belongings from the patient's room is step 13 in the procedure. All three of these steps are part of the discharge procedure for patients leaving the facility.

(103) (B) Any specific instructions for post-discharge care.

The discharge procedure states that a written discharge order should be obtained from the treating physician, which should include any specific instructions for post-discharge care to ensure proper follow-up and continued care.

(104) (C) If the patient requires ongoing medical care or assistance upon discharge, make sure that appropriate arrangements have been made with the relevant home care agency or community health facility.

If the patient requires ongoing medical care or assistance upon discharge, the discharge procedure states that appropriate arrangements should be made with the relevant home care agency or community health facility to ensure that the patient continues to receive the care needed after leaving the hospital.

(105) (A) Persistent cough lasting three or more weeks

Tuberculosis (TB) is a bacterial infection that primarily affects the lungs, but can also affect other parts of the body. The most common symptom of TB is a persistent cough that lasts for more than three weeks, often accompanied by other symptoms such as night sweats, fever, weight loss, and fatigue. Weight gain, increased appetite, and skin rashes are not typically associated with TB.

(106) (B) Annual flu vaccination

The best way to prevent the flu is to get vaccinated each year. The flu vaccine is designed to protect against the influenza viruses that research indicates will be most common during the upcoming season. While other measures like maintaining good hygiene and a healthy lifestyle can help, they are not as effective as the annual flu vaccination. Wearing gloves at all times is not practical and doesn't necessarily prevent the flu, and while Vitamin C and hydration are good for overall health, they're not specific preventative measures against the flu.

(107) (B) If the patient requires ongoing medical care or assistance upon discharge, make sure that appropriate arrangements have been made with the relevant home care agency or community health facility.

The third step in the discharge procedure is to make sure appropriate arrangements have been made with the relevant home care agency or community health facility if the patient requires ongoing medical care or assistance upon discharge.

(108) (B) The comprehensive medication list for the patient.

Prior to discharge, the discharge procedure states that a comprehensive medication list for the patient should be created, including the name, dosage, frequency and any potential side effects or interactions.

(109) (D) Align the medication schedule with the patient's daily routine and lifestyle.

The discharge procedure states that the medication schedule should be aligned with the patient's daily routine and lifestyle. This step is important to ensure the patient takes the medication as prescribed and their health is not negatively impacted.

(110) (B) Hands-on demonstration and written instructions.

The discharge procedure states that hands-on demonstration and written instructions should be provided for self-care procedures or treatments that the patient or the family will perform at home, such as wound care or administering medication.

(111) (C) Pregnant women and individuals with chronic illnesses

While it's recommended that everyone 6 months of age and older should get a flu vaccine every season, it's particularly important for certain groups. Pregnant women, individuals with chronic illnesses like asthma, diabetes, heart or lung disease, as well as those who are immunocompromised are more likely to get severe flu, which can lead to hospitalization or even death. Hence, they are strongly advised to get the flu vaccine annually to protect themselves.

(112) (A) Create a comprehensive medication list for the patient.

The fifth step in the discharge procedure is to create a comprehensive medication list for the patient. This step is important to ensure the patient and the family understand the patient's medication, including the name, dosage, frequency and any potential side effects or interactions.

(113) (C) Reviewing and discussing Mr. Arkin's individualized discharge care plan with him and his family.

In the case of Mr. Arkin, the most important step taken during the discharge process was to review and discuss his individualized discharge care plan with him and his family. This step was crucial to ensure that Mr. Arkin and his family understood his care plan and any updates made during his hospital stay, as well as any instructions for post-discharge care.

(114) (C) Making sure appropriate arrangements have been made with the relevant home care agency or community health facility.

In the case of Mrs. Lewis, who required ongoing medical care after her hospital discharge, the most critical step in the discharge procedure was to make sure appropriate arrangements had been made with the relevant home care agency or community health facility.

(115) (C) Confirming a follow-up appointment with the physician.

The most critical step in Mr. Olivares's discharge was to confirm with the physician. This step was essential to ensure that Mr. Olivares had a scheduled follow-up appointment and was aware of the date, time and location of the appointment.

(116) (A) Obtaining a written discharge order from the treating physician.

This step is critical because it ensures that the hospital staff has a clear understanding of the medical care the patient will require after his discharge and any specific instructions for post-discharge care.

(117) (A) Collect the patient's personal belongings.

The first step a nurse should take when a patient is ready to leave the facility is to collect the patient's personal belongings from the room. This step is important, as it helps ensure that the patient does not leave behind anything of value and that personal belongings are secured and protected.

(118) (B) Patient- and family-centered care is a person-centered approach to health care that values the unique needs and perspectives of patients and their families and emphasizes collaboration and partnership between health care providers, patients and families.

Patient- and family-centered care is a holistic and person-centered approach to health care that values the unique needs, preferences and perspectives of patients and their families.

(119) (C) Valuing the unique needs and perspectives of patients and families.

The respect and dignity principle in patient- and family-centered care places a strong emphasis on listening to and honoring the perspectives and choices of patients and their families.

(120) (C) To promote teamwork and cooperation between all stakeholders in health care.

Collaboration in patient- and family-centered care seeks to create a culture of cooperation between patients, families, health care practitioners and leaders in all aspects of health care. This includes policy, program development, facility design, professional education, research and care delivery.

(121) (A) To ensure that the patient's needs are met throughout the care process.

The main goal of care coordination in health care is to ensure that the patient's needs are met throughout the care process by organizing patient care activities among multiple participants, identifying potential barriers to continuity of care, communicating with other health care providers and agencies and facilitating the transfer of patient information.

(122) (A) Improving the efficiency and accuracy of the process.

The main benefit of implementing automated workflows in the care coordination process is improving the efficiency and accuracy of the process. Automated workflows streamline the coordination process and help minimize errors and delays, making it more efficient and accurate.

(123) (B) Individualized patient care.

The main focus of interprofessional roles and responsibilities in health care is to provide comprehensive patient care by dividing the various tasks and functions among different health care professionals. This includes tasks such as diagnosis, treatment planning, patient education and ongoing care coordination.

(124) (C) Regaining the ability to perform daily activities.

Physical therapists focus on improving the patient's physical strength and mobility, while occupational therapists focus on helping the patient regain the ability to perform daily activities.

(125) (B) Reviewing medication history and making recommendations to the physician.

The pharmacist may review the patient's medication history and make recommendations to the physician while the physician makes the final decision on the appropriate medication.

(126) (D) Case manager.

The social worker may provide emotional support and connect patients with community resources, while the case manager coordinates services and ensures that the patient's care is consistent across different health care settings.

(127) (B) Helping patients recover from injuries or illnesses.

Physical therapists work with occupational therapists to help patients recover from injuries or illnesses. The physical therapist focuses on improving the patient's physical strength and mobility.

(128) (C) To hold back underlying organs or tissues, providing access to the surgical site

A surgical retractor is a surgical instrument used to separate the edges of a surgical incision or wound, or to hold back underlying organs or tissues, so that body parts underneath the incision may be accessed. The usage of a retractor can vastly improve visibility and accessibility during the procedure.

(129) (C) To cut or dissect tissue during surgery

A scalpel is a small, sharp knife that is used in surgeries to make incisions in the skin and other tissues. The scalpel is one of the most crucial tools in a surgeon's toolkit. Different sizes and types of scalpel blades may be used depending on the nature and location of the surgery.

(130) (B) Prevention and wellness.

The first level of care within a continuum of care is prevention and wellness, which includes activities such as health education, screenings and vaccinations that help prevent illness and promote overall health and well-being.

(131) (C) Primary care.

Primary care is provided by a patient's primary care physician or nurse practitioner and includes routine check-ups, screenings and management of common illnesses.

(132) (D) Rehabilitation.

Rehabilitation is focused on helping patients recover from illness or injury and includes services such as physical therapy, occupational therapy and speech therapy.

(133) (B) End-of-life care.

End-of-life care is focused on comfort and support for patients nearing the end of life. This level of care includes hospice care, palliative care and bereavement support for family members.

(134) (D) Long-term care.

Long-term care is provided for patients with chronic conditions that require ongoing management and support. This type of care includes services such as home health care, skilled nursing care and assisted living.

(135) (D) All of the above.

Medical-surgical nurses' main responsibilities include educating the patient about the procedure, assessing the patient's medical history and current condition and ensuring the patient is properly prepared for the procedure.

(136) (C) Provide care to the patient.

Medical-surgical nurses play a critical role in providing care before, during and after surgery. In the postoperative phase, their main focus is on providing care to the patient as they recover from the procedure. This includes monitoring vital signs, managing pain and ensuring the patient is on the path to a successful recovery.

(137) (D) All of the above.

Their responsibilities include monitoring the patient's vital signs, providing support to the surgical team, assisting with positioning the patient, administering medication and preparing the patient for transport to the recovery room.

(138) (A) Monitoring the patient's vital signs.

This includes monitoring the patient's vital signs, such as heart rate, blood pressure and breathing, to assess overall condition and detect any potential problems early on.

(139) (D) All of the above.

Patients with chronic conditions, such as heart failure, COPD and diabetes, as well as those who have recently undergone a surgical procedure or have been discharged from the ICU, are at increased risk for readmission to the hospital. Other factors include poor communication between health care providers, lack of social support and inadequate follow-up care after discharge.

(140) (B) Structure, outcome and process.

The Donabedian model, named after the physician and researcher who formulated it, is a widely recognized framework for assessing and comparing the quality of health care organizations. This model classifies measures used to evaluate quality into three distinct categories: structure, outcome and process.

(141) (D) All of the above.

Examples of structural measures include the utilization of EHRs or medication order entry systems, the proportion of board-certified physicians within an organization and the ratio of providers to patients. Utilizing EHRs and medication order entry systems provides a more efficient and organized way of keeping track of patients' information.

(142) (C) Proportion of patients who receive preventive services.

One example of a process measure is the proportion of patients who receive preventive services, such as cancer screenings or vaccinations.

(143) (C) To evaluate the impact of health care services or interventions on the health status of patients.

These measures provide an understanding of how well the health care service or intervention has performed in improving patient outcomes, such as the mortality rate of patients after a surgical procedure or the rate of complications or infections acquired during hospital stays.

(144) (C) Within the first 48 hours after symptoms start

Explanation: Antiviral drugs work best when started soon after flu illness begins. When treatment is started within two days of becoming sick with flu symptoms, antiviral drugs can lessen fever and flu symptoms, and shorten the time you are sick by about one day. They may also prevent serious flu complications. While it's not a substitute for the flu vaccine, it's a valuable treatment option for individuals who have the flu.

(145) (D) All of the above.

The purpose of documenting nurses' work is to communicate effectively with other members of the health care team; provide information for professionals involved in accreditation, credentialing, legal, regulatory, reimbursement, research and quality activities; and ensure continuity of care.

(146) (B) Accessible, accurate and relevant.

High-quality nursing documentation should be easily accessible to all members of the health care team, as well as those involved in accreditation, credentialing, legal, regulatory, reimbursement, research and quality activities. It should also be accurate, relevant to the patient's condition and care and consistent across all documentation.

(147) (B) Clarity.

Clarity is an important attribute of high-quality nursing documentation, as it ensures that the information is easy to understand and is presented in a straightforward manner.

(148) (B) To reduce medical errors and improve patient care.

EHRs contain a patient's complete medical history, including demographic information, vital signs, medications, allergies, immunizations, laboratory test results and other relevant health information.

(149) (A) Establishing communication protocols.

Downtime procedures aim to minimize the impact of disruptions on patient care. Establishing protocols for how staff will communicate during an outage is one of the steps toward that goal.

(150) (C) A procedure to handle system outages and disruptions to minimize the impact on patient care.

This procedure is planned beforehand and is ready to implement when needed. Staff should be well-educated in the mechanics of the procedure.

Test 3: Questions

(1) An 80-year-old woman is admitted to the medical-surgical unit with a history of falls. What is the most appropriate action for the nurse to take in regard to fall prevention?

(A) Assign the patient to a bed near the exit and limit the patient's mobility.

(B) Assess the patient's fall risk, implement fall prevention strategies and document the assessment and strategies in the patient's chart.

(C) Increase the patient's medication dosage to sedate her and reduce her mobility.

(D) Implement fall prevention strategies only if the patient requests them or if they are deemed necessary by the physician.

(2) Which of the following is an important aspect of medication administration?

(A) Monitoring patients for potential side effects

(B) Understanding the different routes of administration

(C) Proper dosage

(D) All of the above

(3) Which step of the nursing process involves identifying potential health problems based on the information gathered during the assessment step?

(A) Assessment

(B) Diagnosis

(C) Planning

(D) Implementation

(4) Which of the following is not included in the NPSGs for a health care organization?

(A) Improve the accuracy of patient identification.

(B) Enhance communication among caregivers.

(C) Improve the safety of using medications.

(D) Increase patient satisfaction.

(5) A patient is admitted to the hospital with a severe allergic reaction to a medication he had been prescribed. The nurse on duty is tasked with identifying which of the following types of reaction this scenario represents?

(A) Environmental

(B) Equipment

(C) Pharmacological

(D) Human factors

(6) A patient falls in the hospital and suffers a broken hip. The nurse on duty is tasked with identifying which of the following types of risk this scenario represents?

(A) Demographic

(B) Environmental

(C) Economic

(D) Legal and ethical

(7) A patient has just completed surgery. Which tool is important for identifying and addressing potential complications after surgery?

(A) Preoperative assessment

(B) Incident reporting

(C) Continuous quality improvement

(D) Postoperative assessment

(8) A nurse on duty needs to ensure that all necessary steps are taken before, during and after surgery to prevent errors and complications. Which tool should the nurse use?

(A) Preoperative assessment

(B) Incident reporting

(C) Continuous quality improvement

(D) Checklist

(9) What is the purpose of the time-out procedure in surgical settings?

(A) To evaluate the patient's response to anesthesia

(B) To ensure that all necessary steps are taken before, during and after surgery to prevent errors and complications

(C) To confirm the correct patient, procedure and surgical site

(D) To monitor vital signs and pain levels after surgery

(10) What is the primary goal of the Speak Up initiative in health care?

(A) To improve patient satisfaction

(B) To increase communication and participation of patients in care decisions

(C) To reduce health care costs

(D) To improve staff productivity

(11) How does high accountability in health care organizations contribute to a strong patient safety culture?

(A) By promoting transparency and learning from errors

(B) By ensuring all employees understand their roles and responsibilities in ensuring patient safety and holding them accountable for their actions

(C) By fostering a culture of blame and punishment

(D) By setting strict targets and incentives

(12) Why is the just-culture concept important for patient safety culture in health care organizations?

(A) It encourages staff to report errors without fear of retaliation.

(B) It allows for quick resolution of issues.

(C) It promotes a blame-free environment.

(D) It improves the overall patient experience.

(13) What is the main goal of care bundles?

(A) To improve the quality and safety of care

(B) To reduce the cost of care

(C) To increase patient satisfaction

(D) To increase the number of procedures performed

(14) What is the main purpose of a checklist in a care bundle?

(A) To provide a structured approach to care

(B) To guide decision-making

(C) To ensure that all necessary steps are taken before, during and after the procedure or treatment

(D) To reduce complications and cut down costs of the treatment

(15) An example of a checklist in a care bundle for preventing VAP might include _____.

(A) Elevating the head of the bed

(B) Using thrombolytic therapy (clot-busting medication)

(C) Early initiation of rehabilitation

(D) Rapid assessment and diagnosis

(16) An algorithm in a care bundle would typically include _____

(A) Assessing the patient's pain level

(B) Recognizing and activating the emergency medical services

(C) Administering broad-spectrum antibiotics as soon as possible

(D) All of the above

(17) How often are the algorithms in a care bundle reviewed and updated?

(A) Never

(B) Once a year

(C) When new evidence emerges

(D) Every five years

(18) What is the main purpose of patient safety assessment?

(A) To identify and evaluate potential hazards that could harm patients in a health care setting

(B) To improve the patient care process

(C) To share information about identified hazards with staff, patients and other stakeholders

(D) To manage the assessment and reporting of safety issues

(19) What is the last step in the process of patient safety assessment?

(A) Identification of hazards

(B) Evaluation of risks

(C) Control and prevention

(D) Monitoring and evaluation

(20) A health care facility is experiencing a high number of incidents related to medication errors. The facility wants to implement a patient safety assessment to identify the root cause of the problem and prevent future incidents. What is the first step in conducting the patient safety assessment?

(A) Evaluation of risks

(B) Control and prevention

(C) Identification of hazards

(D) Communication and education

(21) What is the main goal of patient safety reporting?

(A) To identify problems and issues related to patient safety as soon as possible

(B) To submit reports of specific incidents or adverse events

(C) To investigate the underlying causes of incidents or adverse events

(D) To receive patient complaints

(22) What is the difference between incident reporting and near-miss reporting?

(A) Incident reporting involves reporting incidents that have already caused harm, while near-miss reporting involves reporting incidents that have the potential to cause harm.

(B) Incident reporting involves submitting reports of specific incidents or adverse events, while near-miss reporting involves investigating the underlying causes of incidents or adverse events.

(C) Incident reporting involves identifying ways to prevent incidents from happening again in the future, while near-miss reporting involves identifying ways to prevent incidents from happening in the first place.

(D) Incident reporting is mandatory, while near-miss reporting is optional.

(23) Why is root cause analysis important in patient safety reporting?

(A) It helps identify the underlying causes of incidents or adverse events.

(B) It allows health care organizations to track and analyze data on incidents and near-misses.

(C) It helps organizations identify ways to prevent incidents from happening again in the future.

(D) All of the above.

(24) A health care facility is experiencing a high number of incidents related to medication errors. The facility wants to implement a patient safety reporting process to identify the root cause of the problem and prevent future incidents. What are the steps the facility should take in conducting the patient safety reporting process?

(A) Root cause analysis, incident reporting, near-miss reporting, patient complaints

(B) Root cause analysis, incident reporting, patient complaints, near-miss reporting

(C) Incident reporting, near-miss reporting, root cause analysis, patient complaints

(D) Patient complaints, incident reporting, root cause analysis, near-miss reporting

(25) What is the first step a medical-surgical nurse should take if he suspects a patient is a victim of abuse?

(A) Report the suspected abuse to the police or child protective services.

(B) Document the suspected abuse in the patient's medical record.

(C) Provide emotional support and information to the patient.

(D) Inform the supervisor or designated abuse reporting contact.

(26) What should the medical-surgical nurse be aware of when reporting suspected abuse?

(A) Reporting laws and regulations in the area

(B) Providing emotional support and information to the patient

(C) Sharing available resources and options, such as safe housing and counseling services

(D) All of the above

(27) A health care provider wants to identify and understand the social factors impacting a patient's health. What is the first step the provider should take?

(A) Assessing patients for SDOH during clinical encounters

(B) Collecting data and analyzing it to identify patterns and trends

(C) Collaborating with community-based organizations or other partners

(D) Making appropriate referrals to community resources

(28) A health care provider is examining a patient and suspects that she may be a victim of human trafficking. What is the first step the provider should take?

(A) Inform the supervisor or designated trafficking reporting contact.

(B) Report to the appropriate authorities, such as police or federal agencies.

(C) Provide emotional support and information to the patient about the available resources and options.

(D) Maintain the patient's confidentiality.

(29) What is a process that helps identify the underlying cause of an incident or problem?

(A) Safety rounds

(B) Safety huddles

(C) Root Cause Analysis (RCA)

(D) Failure Mode and Effects Analysis (FMEA)

(30) What is a process that helps identify potential failure modes in a process or system and assess the potential consequences of those failure modes?

(A) Safety rounds

(B) Safety huddles

(C) Root Cause Analysis (RCA)

(D) Failure Mode and Effects Analysis (FMEA)

(31) What is a method that involves physically walking through the workplace and looking for potential hazards or unsafe conditions?

(A) Safety rounds

(B) Safety huddles

(C) Root Cause Analysis (RCA)

(D) Failure Mode and Effects Analysis (FMEA)

(32) What is a method that involves a brief, daily meeting to discuss safety issues and identify and address any concerns?

(A) Safety rounds

(B) Safety huddles

(C) Root Cause Analysis (RCA)

(D) Failure Mode and Effects Analysis (FMEA)

(33) Which method is used to identify potential hazards or unsafe conditions and take steps to eliminate them?

(A) Safety rounds

(B) Safety huddles

(C) Root Cause Analysis (RCA)

(D) Risk assessment

(34) According to OSHA guidelines, what is the appropriate action for an employee who notices a sharp object on the floor of the workplace?

(A) Do not report it, as it may cause inconvenience to colleagues.

(B) Leave it where it is and hope someone else will pick it up.

(C) Pick it up and dispose of it in the designated sharps container.

(D) Ignore it and continue with his work.

(35) Which of the following best describes the purpose of airborne precautions?

(A) To minimize contact with pathogens that are spread through the air in close contact and affect the respiratory system or mucous membranes

(B) To reduce the risk of transmission of pathogens that are acquired through direct or indirect contact, particularly MDROs

(C) To prevent the spread of organisms that can cause infection over long distances when suspended in the air

(D) To prevent the spread of pathogens that are spread through the air in close contact

(36) Which pathogens are typically spread through droplets and require the use of droplet precautions?

(A) HIV and hepatitis C

(B) Tuberculosis and salmonella

(C) Influenza and pertussis

(D) Herpes and HPV

(37) What best describes the purpose of contact precautions?

(A) To reduce the risk of transmission of pathogens that are acquired through direct or indirect contact, specifically MDROs

(B) To reduce the risk of transmission of pathogens that are acquired through respiratory droplets

(C) To reduce the risk of transmission of pathogens that are acquired through food or water

(D) To reduce the risk of transmission of pathogens that are acquired through contact with animals

(38) What is a recommended infection-control measure for preventing the spread of germs on frequently touched surfaces and medical equipment?

(A) Using UV light to disinfect surfaces

(B) Wearing gloves while performing procedures that have a risk of exposure to bodily fluids or contaminated surfaces

(C) Using proper decontamination techniques, such as cleaning and disinfecting

(D) Regularly screening employees for symptoms of infectious diseases and requiring them to stay home if they are sick

(39) What is a recommended infection-control measure for preventing the spread of infection to other patients or health care workers?

(A) Using proper decontamination techniques, such as cleaning and disinfecting

(B) Wearing gloves while performing procedures that have a risk of exposure to bodily fluids or contaminated surfaces

(C) Implementing isolation protocols for patients with contagious illnesses

(D) Regularly screening employees for symptoms of infectious diseases and requiring them to stay home if they are sick

(40) A patient has been diagnosed with a contagious illness and requires isolation to prevent the spread of infection to other patients and health care workers. Which of the following actions should be taken to properly implement isolation protocols for this patient?

(A) Allow the patient to leave the hospital and self-isolate at home.

(B) Place the patient in a room with other patients who are also infected with the same illness.

(C) Place the patient in a private room with a bathroom and limit the number of health care workers who enter the room.

(D) Place the patient in a shared room with no special precautions.

(41) A surgical procedure is being performed. Which action should be taken to properly implement strategies for preventing SSIs?

(A) Health care workers should perform hand hygiene with soap and water or an alcohol-based hand sanitizer only after the procedure.

(B) Health care workers should wear visibly dirty gloves, gowns and masks during the procedure.

(C) Prophylactic antibiotics should only be administered to patients in certain cases.

(D) Health care workers should perform hand hygiene with soap and water or an alcohol-based hand sanitizer before and after each patient contact.

(42) A patient in a health care facility has been diagnosed with an MDRO infection. Which action is considered the most effective in preventing the spread of the infection in the health care facility?

(A) Implementing a wait-and-see approach before taking any action

(B) Isolating the infected patient in a separate room without implementing any infection-control measures

(C) Implementing infection-control measures, such as proper hand hygiene, use of PPE, appropriate cleaning and disinfection of health care environments, and active surveillance for the presence of MDROs to identify and isolate infected individuals

(D) Restricting the use of antibiotics and other antimicrobial agents in the health care facility

(43) What is the main goal of antimicrobial stewardship programs in relation to MDROs?

(A) To promote the use of broad-spectrum antibiotics

(B) To encourage unnecessary antibiotic use

(C) To promote the appropriate use of antibiotics, including the use of narrow-spectrum antibiotics and the avoidance of unnecessary antibiotic use

(D) To increase the spread of MDROs

(44) What is the specific method used in regular feedback and audits of antibiotic prescribing practices in an antimicrobial stewardship program to track the emergence of antibiotic-resistant organisms?

(A) Monitoring the number of prescriptions written

(B) Evaluating the effectiveness of interventions

(C) Keeping a record of resistance patterns

(D) Tracking the spread of antibiotic-resistant organisms using molecular epidemiology techniques

(45) What is the stage of medication administration where errors are more likely to occur?

(A) Medication administration to the patient

(B) The ordering and preparing phase

(C) The post-assessment of the patient

(D) Medication storage

(46) Why are parenteral medications considered high-alert medications?

(A) They have a high potential for abuse.

(B) They are expensive.

(C) They have a potential for significant harm when used in error.

(D) They are difficult to administer.

(47) What is a common source of errors during medication administration?

(A) Miscommunication between health care staff

(B) Incorrectly labeling or storing medications

(C) Lack of proper equipment or technology

(D) All of the above

(48) Which step can be taken to minimize the risk of medication errors in high-alert medications?

(A) Increasing the frequency of medication administration

(B) Using error-prone abbreviations or symbols

(C) Implementing strict protocols for medication preparation and administration

(D) Ignoring the potential consequences of errors

(49) How often should health care providers check in with patients to ensure they understand and are following the medication regimen correctly?

(A) Once a week

(B) Once a month

(C) During regular check-ups or follow-up appointments

(D) None of the above

(50) What is the definition of polypharmacy?

(A) The use of a single medication

(B) The use of multiple medications

(C) The use of unnecessary or inappropriate medications

(D) The use of herbal products or supplements

(51) Which factor can affect patient satisfaction in health care?

(A) The cost of treatment

(B) The responsiveness of health care staff

(C) The availability of technology

(D) The availability of public transportation

(52) What is the most common method used to gather feedback from patients regarding their satisfaction with health care services?

(A) Personal interviews

(B) Surveys

(C) Focus groups

(D) Online reviews

(53) What is the primary purpose of The Joint Commission's guidelines on patient satisfaction measurement and improvement?

(A) To provide health care organizations with a benchmark for quality and safety of care

(B) To increase the number of patients that visit health care organizations

(C) To promote patient satisfaction in a nonmedical way

(D) To decrease patient complaints

(54) What is a key aspect of The Joint Commission's guidelines on patient satisfaction measurement and improvement?

(A) Administering standardized patient satisfaction surveys

(B) Providing financial incentives for patients who are satisfied with their care

(C) Offering discounts for patients who provide positive feedback

(D) Improving the overall quality of life for patients

(55) What is the goal of gathering feedback from patients through standardized patient satisfaction surveys per The Joint Commission's guidelines?

(A) To reduce patient complaints

(B) To improve the patient experience

(C) To increase staff productivity

(D) To identify areas in need of improvement

(56) How does using patient satisfaction data in performance evaluations for individual providers and staff help improve patient satisfaction according to The Joint Commission's guidelines?

(A) By sharing the results of the patient satisfaction survey with staff

(B) By providing a mechanism for patients to file complaints and grievances

(C) By holding staff accountable for the care they provide

(D) By collecting and analyzing patient satisfaction data on a regular basis

(57) What is the main purpose of getting a second opinion for a patient?

(A) To provide a more accurate diagnosis

(B) To provide a quicker treatment

(C) To reduce the cost of treatment

(D) To increase confidence and reduce anxiety

(58) What is the most important piece of information for a nurse to know when referring a patient for a second opinion?

(A) The patient's previous diagnoses

(B) The patient's current test results

(C) The patient's insurance coverage

(D) The patient's level of understanding and ability to participate in decision-making

(59) A 45-year-old patient named Mary has been experiencing chronic back pain for the past year. She has already seen several health care providers and has received multiple treatments, including physical therapy, pain medications and spinal injections. However, none of these treatments have provided lasting relief.

Mary is now seeking a second opinion on her condition and treatment options.

What information should the nurse collecting information for Mary's second opinion appointment gather to ensure the specialist has the necessary information to make an informed decision?

(A) Mary's current symptoms and concerns

(B) Mary's current test results and imaging studies

(C) Any previous treatment options that have been tried and the results of those treatments

(D) All of the above

(60) What is the first step in the service recovery process?

(A) Apologizing to the patient

(B) Providing compensation to the patient

(C) Identifying the problem that has occurred

(D) Fixing the problem

(61) How can a sincere apology impact the negative effects of a poor patient experience?

(A) It makes the patient more upset.

(B) It does not have an impact on the patient.

(C) It shows the patient that the health care organization recognizes and takes responsibility for the problem.

(D) It makes the patient feel ignored.

(62) What is the difference between a complaint and a grievance in the health care setting?

(A) Complaints are minor issues related to room cleanliness, whereas grievances are serious issues related to patient care or Medicare billing.

(B) Complaints are serious issues related to patient care or Medicare billing, whereas grievances are minor issues related to room cleanliness.

(C) Complaints pertain to issues with staff performance, whereas grievances pertain to issues with facility policies.

(D) Complaints and grievances are the same thing.

(63) Who can file a grievance in the health care setting?

(A) Only the patient

(B) Only the staff present at the time of the incident

(C) Only the patient's representative

(D) Both the patient and the representative

(64) Which of the following laboratory values indicates a potential complication of diabetic ketoacidosis (DKA)?

(A) Increased blood glucose levels

(B) Decreased serum potassium levels

(C) Elevated blood pH

(D) Low urine ketone levels

(65) A patient with heart failure presents with shortness of breath, crackles on auscultation, and edema in the lower extremities. Which medication would be most appropriate for managing these symptoms?

(A) Loop diuretics

(B) Beta-blockers

(C) Calcium channel blockers

(D) Angiotensin-converting enzyme (ACE) inhibitors

(66) Which of the following is a risk factor for the development of deep vein thrombosis (DVT)?

(A) Hypertension

(B) Hyperglycemia

(C) Obesity

(D) Hypothyroidism

(67) A patient is admitted with suspected appendicitis. Which assessment finding would be most concerning and indicate possible rupture of the appendix?

(A) Rebound tenderness in the right lower quadrant

(B) Nausea and vomiting

(C) Increased pain with movement

(D) Fever and chills

(68) A patient with chronic obstructive pulmonary disease (COPD) is prescribed long-term oxygen therapy. Which assessment finding would indicate the need for adjustment of oxygen therapy?

(A) Increased respiratory rate

(B) Decreased oxygen saturation

(C) Dry cough

(D) Elevated blood pressure

(69) A patient with a myocardial infarction (MI) is displaying signs of worsening heart failure. Which of the following symptoms would be most concerning?

(A) Persistent cough

(B) Shortness of breath

(C) Increased urine output

(D) Weight loss

(70) In a patient with Addison's disease, what would you expect to find upon assessment?

(A) Hypernatremia and hypokalemia

(B) Hypernatremia and hyperkalemia

(C) Hyponatremia and hyperkalemia

(D) Hyponatremia and hypokalemia

(71) What are the most important interventions for a patient with acute pancreatitis?

(A) Frequent feeding and administration of insulin

(B) Pain management and NPO (nil per os/nothing by mouth)

(C) High protein diet and diuretics

(D) Administration of antibiotics and regular exercise

(72) A patient with Guillain-Barré syndrome (GBS) begins to exhibit difficulty with speech and swallowing. This could be an indication of:

(A) Impending full recovery

(B) Normal disease progression

(C) Worsening or ascending paralysis

(D) Beginning of relapse

(73) Which intervention is most important in the care of a patient with a suspected pulmonary embolism (PE)?

(A) Ambulation to prevent further clot formation

(B) Administration of a diuretic to decrease fluid volume

(C) Oxygen therapy and anticoagulation as prescribed

(D) Frequent chest physiotherapy to improve lung function

(74) What is cultural competence in health care?

(A) Recognizing and respecting cultural differences

(B) Providing care that is sensitive to the cultural and linguistic needs of patients from diverse backgrounds

(C) Knowing all the cultural practices of every patient

(D) Being familiar with the languages spoken by patients

(75) Which of the following principles from the NCSBN guidelines is the most crucial for ensuring that nurses are providing culturally and linguistically appropriate care to their patients?

(A) Respect for diversity

(B) Cultural humility

(C) Language access

(D) Ongoing learning

(76) A nurse is assigned to take care of a patient from a different culture who speaks a language that the nurse does not understand. The patient is experiencing severe pain and is unable to communicate his symptoms effectively. What should the nurse do to provide culturally and linguistically appropriate care to this patient in accordance with the NCSBN guidelines?

(A) Call in a language specialist to interpret for the patient.

(B) Ignore the patient's cultural background and proceed with the usual pain management procedure.

(C) Use gestures and expressions to try to understand the patient's symptoms.

(D) Inform the patient that he needs to speak English in order to receive proper medical care.

(77) What is the most common way for a patient who is deaf or hard of hearing to communicate with health care providers?

(A) Written language

(B) Sign languages

(C) Spoken language

(D) Facial expressions

(78) What is the role of health care providers in ensuring that patients with cultural and linguistic needs receive appropriate care?

(A) Providing only sign language interpreters for deaf or hard-of-hearing patients

(B) Relying on family members or friends to interpret for patients who speak languages other than the dominant language in the health care setting

(C) Providing a variety of communication methods, including interpreter services and translated materials, to accommodate the cultural and linguistic needs of all patients

(D) Providing written materials only in the dominant language of the health care setting

(79) What is the most common solution for patients who speak a language other than the dominant language in a health care setting to communicate with health care providers and understand their health conditions and treatment options?

(A) Sign languages

(B) Oral languages in written form

(C) Written languages

(D) Interpreter services or translated materials in the preferred language

(80) A patient is admitted with suspected pulmonary embolism. Which diagnostic test is most commonly used to confirm the diagnosis?

(A) Chest X-ray

(B) Electrocardiogram (ECG)

(C) Pulmonary angiography

(D) D-dimer blood test

(81) A patient with chronic kidney disease is at risk for developing metabolic acidosis. Which arterial blood gas (ABG) value would be consistent with metabolic acidosis?

(A) pH 7.48, PaCO2 42 mmHg, HCO3- 26 mEq/L

(B) pH 7.32, PaCO2 48 mmHg, HCO3- 22 mEq/L

(C) pH 7.42, PaCO2 38 mmHg, HCO3- 24 mEq/L

(D) pH 7.52, PaCO2 30 mmHg, HCO3- 20 mEq/L

(82) A patient with a history of peptic ulcer disease is prescribed a proton pump inhibitor (PPI). How does a PPI exert its therapeutic effect?

(A) By neutralizing gastric acid

(B) By increasing gastric motility

(C) By blocking histamine receptors

(D) By inhibiting gastric acid secretion

(83) Which of the following is a common complication associated with prolonged immobility in hospitalized patients?

(A) Hypernatremia

(B) Hypokalemia

(C) Deep vein thrombosis (DVT)

(D) Hyperglycemia

(D) To be aware of potential biases and actively seek out opportunities to learn about different cultures

(84) What is implicit bias?

(A) Conscious attitudes or stereotypes toward certain groups of people

(B) Unconscious attitudes or stereotypes toward certain groups of people

(C) Attitudes and beliefs that people are aware of and can control

(D) Attitudes and beliefs that people are not aware of and cannot control

(85) Implicit bias can lead to _____.

(A) Improved quality of care for patients

(B) Disparities in the quality of care that patients receive

(C) Increased trust and communication between health care providers and patients

(D) No impact on the quality of care that patients receive

(86) Which role do health care organizations play in reducing the effects of implicit bias in health care?

(A) No role

(B) Providing training for health care providers on cultural competence

(C) Implementing policies and procedures to promote diversity, equity and inclusion

(D) Developing a patient-centered approach and actively seeking out diverse perspectives

(87) Dr. Rodriguez has noticed that the clinic she works in tends to treat patients of a certain racial or ethnic group differently than other patients. This has led to lower-quality care and a lack of trust and communication between the doctor and these patients. What steps can the doctor take to reduce the effects of implicit bias?

(A) Refrain from forming any opinions or stereotypes about patients.

(B) Implement policies and procedures to promote diversity, equity and inclusion.

(C) Develop a patient-centered approach and actively seek out diverse perspectives.

(D) Receive training on cultural competence and awareness of her own biases.

(88) What is one of a nurse's key responsibilities in health maintenance?

(A) Administering medications

(B) Educating patients and families about healthy behaviors

(C) Cleaning equipment

(D) Operating surgical instruments

(89) What is one of the steps in health maintenance that a nurse can take to prevent the spread of infectious diseases?

(A) Screen for common diseases

(B) Assess the patient's health status

(C) Implement infection-control measures

(D) Administer vaccinations

(90) What is one way a nurse can encourage patient self-management and self-care?

(A) Screen for common diseases

(B) Assess the patient's health status

(C) Implement infection-control measures

(D) Provide education and resources to patients and families

(91) In what ways can nurses support the health maintenance of a patient with heart disease?

(A) Administer vaccinations and educate patients on healthy behaviors.

(B) Implement infection-control measures and address behavioral health needs.

(C) Assess and address the patient's health status, screen for common diseases and refer for follow-up care.

(D) Encourage patient self-management and self-care and update knowledge and skills through continuing education.

(92) The ANA encourages nurses to educate patients and the public about
_____.

(A) What drugs to take

(B) Proper nutrition and early disease detection

(C) The benefits of vaccinations

(D) The importance of PPE use

(93) What does the ANA support as a safe and effective way to prevent the spread of infectious diseases?

(A) Regular screenings and early detection

(B) The use of PPE

(C) Vaccination

(D) Isolation for five days

(94) The ANA encourages nurses to advocate for _____.

(A) Access to affordable health care, healthy food options and safe housing

(B) Proper nutrition and adequate sleep

(C) The benefits of early disease detection

(D) The importance of vaccination

(95) A patient with heart failure is prescribed an angiotensin-converting enzyme (ACE) inhibitor. What is the primary therapeutic effect of ACE inhibitors in heart failure?

(A) Increased heart rate

(B) Decreased blood pressure

(C) Reduced fluid retention

(D) Enhanced myocardial contractility

(96) What is the relationship between health literacy and the ability to make informed decisions about one's health?

(A) Health literacy is the cause of making informed decisions about one's health.

(B) Health literacy is the result of making informed decisions about one's health.

(C) Health literacy is a necessary condition for making informed decisions about one's health.

(D) Making informed decisions about one's health has no relationship with health literacy.

(97) What role do nurses play in improving health literacy levels among patients?

(A) They assess patients' health literacy level and communicate by using clear and simple language.

(B) They provide written materials that are easy to read and understand.

(C) They encourage patients to participate in their care and ask questions.

(D) All of the above.

(98) In a scenario where a patient has limited health literacy, what is the most appropriate approach for a nurse to take to communicate with a patient and ensure he understands his health information?

(A) Speak to the patient using medical jargon and complex terms.

(B) Provide the patient with written materials that are difficult to understand.

(C) Use clear, simple language and provide written materials that are easy to read and understand.

(D) Encourage the patient to rely on a family member or caregiver to understand the health information.

(99) In a scenario where a patient is skeptical about the benefits of vaccines, what is the role of a nurse in advocating for the use of vaccines?

(A) Agree with the patient's skepticism and avoid discussing the use of vaccines.

(B) Provide the patient with written materials that highlight the dangers of vaccines.

(C) Provide the patient with balanced and accurate information about the benefits and risks of vaccines.

(D) Persuade the patient to get vaccinated.

(100) What is the primary component of the patient education process that ensures its effectiveness and success?

(A) The use of technology

(B) The quality of the written materials provided

(C) The continuous assessment and adaptation of teaching strategies

(D) The length of time spent in patient teaching

(101) What is the main goal of original individualized care in nursing?

(A) To provide one-size-fits-all care to all patients

(B) To respect the patient's cultural and personal values

(C) To recognize the patient as a unique individual

(D) To provide care based on the nurse's experiences

(102) Which of the following is an example of a standard precaution for infection control?

(A) Wearing gloves during patient care

(B) Disinfecting surfaces with an appropriate cleaner

(C) Wearing a gown and mask in an isolation room

(D)Administering antibiotics to a patient with an infection

(103) A patient is admitted to the hospital with multiple chronic conditions and is in need of coordinated care from multiple health care professionals. Which of the following approaches to care is most likely to be effective in meeting the patient's needs?

(A) A single health care professional providing care

(B) A group of health care professionals with the same area of expertise working together

(C) A group of health care professionals with different areas of expertise working together

(D) A group of health care professionals providing care without coordination

(104) The nursing staff is having difficulty communicating with the physician team about the care of a particular patient. What is an effective method for promoting nurse-physician collaboration in this scenario?

(A) Ignore the communication issues.

(B) Encourage competition between the health care professionals.

(C) Schedule regular times for the nurse and physician team to meet and discuss the patient's care.

(D) Promote a hierarchical approach to patient care.

(105) What is the main goal of interprofessional rounding?

(A) To improve communication between health care professionals

(B) To provide patients with the most appropriate treatment

(C) To identify potential issues before they become major problems

(D) All of the above

(106) What types of health care professionals typically participate in interprofessional rounding?

(A) Only physicians

(B) Only nurses

(C) Physicians, nurses, social workers and other members of the health care team

(D) Only social workers

(107) During interprofessional rounding, the health care team discovers that a patient's medication regimen is causing adverse effects. What should be the team's next step?

(A) Continue the medication regimen as prescribed.

(B) Consult with the patient's primary physician to make adjustments to the medication regimen.

(C) Discontinue the medication without consulting the physician.

(D) None of the above.

(108) During interprofessional rounding, a patient's care plan needs to be updated to reflect changes in his condition. Who is responsible for updating the care plan?

(A) The interprofessional team as a whole

(B) The patient's primary physician

(C) The nurse responsible for the patient's care

(D) The entire health care team, including the patient and his family

(109) How often do interprofessional rounds typically take place in a health care facility?

(A) Monthly

(B) Hourly

(C) Daily or weekly

(D) Irregularly

(110) What is one of the ways that patients' lack of understanding can negatively impact the health care system?

(A) By reducing the efficiency of referral staff

(B) By increasing trust in the health care system

(C) By leading to confusion, frustration and a lack of trust in the health care system

(D) By improving patient outcomes

(111) What is a specific action that can be taken to achieve coordinated care in primary care practices?

(A) Identifying and assigning roles and responsibilities among health care providers

(B) Improving health care delivery

(C) Ensuring patient autonomy and self-care

(D) Evaluating patient needs and objectives

(112) What is a broad care coordination approach in primary care practices?

(A) Regularly assessing progress

(B) Managing medications

(C) Improving health care delivery

(D) Encouraging patient autonomy and self-care

(113) What is a specific action to achieve coordinated care in primary care practices?

(A) Facilitating smooth transitions of care

(B) Ensuring teamwork among health care providers

(C) Implementing management programs

(D) Ensuring medication management

(114) What is a broad care coordination approach in primary care practices?

(A) Health information technology

(B) Improving health care delivery

(C) Encouraging patient autonomy and self-care

(D) Regularly assessing progress

(115) What is the main goal of collaborative problem-solving in health care?

(A) To improve communication between health care providers

(B) To monitor staff compliance

(C) To develop solutions to address patient care issues

(D) To track the number of medication errors

(116) What is an example of a task performed during collaborative problem-solving in health care?

(A) Tracking the number of medication errors

(B) Implementing a standardized communication protocol

(C) Redesigning the labeling system for medications

(D) None of the above

(117) Which of the following types of resources can provide information on public health issues and outbreaks, as well as resources for patient education and vaccination programs in the community?

(A) Home health agencies

(B) Support groups

(C) Public health departments

(D) Community centers

(118) What is the purpose of community health clinics in the community?

(A) To provide nursing, therapy and other health services to patients in their homes

(B) To provide a wide range of services for the community, such as health screenings, fitness classes and educational programs

(C) To provide primary care and other health services, such as vaccinations and screenings, to people in the community

(D) To provide assistance with things like housing, food and transportation

(119) Which of the following situations may justify the use of physical restraints in a patient?

(A) The patient is non-compliant with care instructions

(B) The patient is frequently asking for assistance

(C) The patient is at risk of harm to self due to confusion or agitation

(D) The patient has refused to eat their meal

(120) When caring for a patient in restraints, how often should a nurse check on the patient's circulation, mobility, and comfort?

(A) Every 4 hours

(B) Once per shift

(C) Every 2 hours

(D) Only at the beginning and end of the shift

(121) What is the first action a nurse should take if they suspect an infiltration of an IV site?

(A) Administer a vasodilator at the site

(B) Apply a warm compress to the site

(C) Immediately remove the IV catheter

(D) Increase the rate of IV fluid administration

(122) When preparing to start an IV on a patient, what is the most appropriate vein selection consideration?

(A) The largest vein available

(B) A vein in the non-dominant arm

(C) A vein that is straight and feels bouncy when palpated

(D) A vein that is superficial and easily visible

(123) What is the goal of the plan the nurse develops for Mr. Smith after his hip replacement surgery?

(A) To evaluate Mr. Smith's physical limitations and conditions

(B) To help Mr. Smith regain or maintain his mobility

(C) To monitor Mr. Smith's progress and adjust the plan as needed

(D) All of the above

(124) What is the purpose of the TUG test?

(A) To measure a patient's ability to perform basic activities of daily living

(B) To assess a patient's risk of falling

(C) To measure a patient's balance and stability

(D) None of the above

(125) What does the BBS test measure?

(A) A patient's ability to perform functional activities

(B) A patient's balance, stability and ability to perform functional activities

(C) A patient's lower body strength and muscle function

(D) None of the above

(126) What is the purpose of the Barthel Index of Activities of Daily Living?

(A) To measure a patient's ability to perform basic activities of daily living

(B) To assess a patient's risk of falling

(C) To measure a patient's ability to reach forward while maintaining balance

(D) All of the above

(127) Which of the following tests measures a patient's ability to stand up from a seated position and sit back down again?

(A) The TUG test

(B) The FTSST test

(C) The BBS test

(D) The Barthel Index of Activities of Daily Living

(128) What is the purpose of the Functional Reach Test?

(A) To assess a patient's balance, stability and ability to perform functional activities

(B) To measure a patient's ability to reach forward while maintaining balance

(C) To measure a patient's ability to perform basic activities of daily living

(D) To assess a patient's risk of falling

(129) Which test measures a patient's ability to perform basic activities of daily living?

(A) The TUG test

(B) The FTSST test

(C) The BBS test

(D) The Barthel Index of Activities of Daily Living

(130) Which of the following tests measures a patient's ability to stand up from a seated position, walk a short distance and return to a seated position?

(A) The TUG test

(B) The FTSST test

(C) The BBS test

(D) The Barthel Index of Activities of Daily Living

(131) Which of the following tests measures a patient's balance, stability and ability to perform functional activities?

(A) The TUG test

(B) The FTSST test

(C) The BBS test

(D) The Barthel Index of Activities of Daily Living

(132) Which of the following tests would a medical professional use to assess a patient's lower body strength and muscle function after a knee replacement surgery?

(A) The TUG test

(B) The FTSST test

(C) The BBS test

(D) The Barthel Index of Activities of Daily Living

(133) Which of the following tests would a medical professional use to assess a patient's risk of falling?

(A) The TUG test

(B) The FTSST test

(C) The BBS test

(D) The Barthel Index of Activities of Daily Living

(134) Which of the following tests would a medical professional use to assess a patient's ability to perform basic activities of daily living, such as bathing, dressing and toileting?

(A) The TUG test

(B) The FTSST test

(C) The BBS test

(D) The Barthel Index of Activities of Daily Living

(135) Which of the following tests would a medical professional use to assess a patient's balance, stability and ability to perform functional activities, such as reaching, turning and stepping?

(A) The TUG test

(B) The FTSST test

(C) The BBS test

(D) The Barthel Index of Activities of Daily Living

(136) A grade of 3 on the Functional Mobility Scale (FMS) indicates a _____.

(A) Patient is unable to move and requires full assistance

(B) Patient is able to move but requires significant assistance

(C) Patient is able to move but requires moderate assistance

(D) Patient is able to move with minimal assistance

(137) A grade of 1 on FMS indicates a _____.

(A) Patient is unable to move and requires full assistance

(B) Patient is able to move but requires significant assistance

(C) Patient is able to move but requires moderate assistance

(D) Patient is able to move with minimal assistance

(138) A grade of 2 on the FMS indicates _____.

(A) Patient is unable to move and requires full assistance

(B) Patient is able to move but requires significant assistance

(C) Patient is able to move but requires moderate assistance

(D) Patient is able to move with minimal assistance

(139) A grade of 4 on the FMS indicates a _____.

(A) Patient is unable to move and requires full assistance

(B) Patient is able to move but requires significant assistance

(C) Patient is able to move but requires moderate assistance

(D) Patient is able to move with minimal assistance

(140) A grade of 0 on the FMS indicates _____.

(A) Patient is unable to move and requires full assistance

(B) Patient is able to move but requires significant assistance

(C) Patient is able to move but requires moderate assistance

(D) Patient is able to move with minimal assistance

(141) A patient has recently had a stroke and is unable to stand or walk without assistance. His grade on the FMS is _____.

(A) 0

(B) 1

(C) 2

(D) 4

(142) A patient has recently recovered from a broken leg and has been doing physical therapy to regain mobility. Her grade on the FMS is _____.

(A) 0

(B) 1

(C) 2

(D) 4

(143) Which grade on the FMS best describes a patient who can walk with a walker but requires someone to be with him for safety?

(A) 0

(B) 1

(C) 2

(D) 3

(144) A patient has been bedridden for a few months due to a serious illness. Her grade on the FMS is _____.

(A) 0

(B) 1

(C) 2

(D) 4

(145) What is the main goal of physical therapy in the case of a patient who has recently had hip replacement surgery?

(A) To manage pain and reduce inflammation

(B) To improve posture and body mechanics

(C) To provide comprehensive evaluation and develop a treatment plan

(D) To improve stability and reduce the risk of falls

(146) How often are physical therapy sessions typically scheduled for a patient recovering from hip surgery?

(A) Once a week

(B) Twice a week

(C) Three times a week

(D) Four times a week

(147) What does the nurse typically do when conducting a health history assessment?

(A) Review the patient's medical history and current symptoms.

(B) Review laboratory results and medical records from other health care providers.

(C) Ask family members or caregivers for information about the patient's health history.

(D) All of the above.

(148) What is the first step that a nurse typically takes when conducting a health history assessment?

(A) Review medical records and laboratory results.

(B) Talk with family members or caregivers.

(C) Ask the patient about medical history and current symptoms.

(D) Obtain information from other health care providers.

(149) What is the first step of the discharge procedure?

(A) Obtain a written discharge order from the treating physician.

(B) Before the day of discharge, notify the patient and their designated family or caregivers of the anticipated discharge date and time.

(C) Prior to discharge, review and discuss the patient's individualized discharge care plan.

(D) Collect the patient's personal belongings from the room.

(150) What is the purpose of creating a comprehensive medication list for the patient?

(A) To perform a final check of the patient's vital signs

(B) To retrieve any personal belongings or valuables that the patient had left in the facility's safe

(C) To review any self-care procedures or treatments that the patient or the family will need to perform at home

(D) To promote compliance and prevent any improper administration of medications

Test 3: Answers & Explanations

(1) (B) Assess the patient's fall risk, implement fall prevention strategies and document the assessment and strategies in the patient's chart.

Implement fall prevention strategies and document them to ensure continuity of care and the patient's safety. This is the most appropriate action for the nurse to take in regard to fall prevention for this patient.

(2) (D) All of the above.

This includes understanding the different routes of administration, as well as the proper dosage. Monitoring patients for potential side effects and interactions of medications is crucial in preventing medication errors and ensuring patient safety. All of these factors are important to consider to ensure the safe administration of medication to patients.

(3) (B) Diagnosis.

Diagnosis is the second step. It involves identifying potential health problems based on the information gathered during assessment. This includes formulating a diagnosis statement that includes the problem, the cause and related symptoms. The diagnoses are then organized for easy planning and implementation of care.

(4) (D) Increase patient satisfaction.

The NPSGs include goals such as improving the accuracy of patient identification; enhancing communication among caregivers; improving the safety of using medications; reducing the risk of infections associated with medical care; protecting every patient from potential harm from falls; and identifying, resolving and preventing adverse events and health care-related pressure ulcers.

(5) (C) Pharmacological.

These types of reactions include risks associated with medications, such as adverse drug reactions, medication errors and drug interactions.

(6) (B) Environmental.

These types of risks include risks associated with the physical environment, such as falls, infections and exposure to hazardous materials.

(7) (D) Postoperative assessment.

A postoperative assessment includes monitoring the patient's vital signs, pain levels and wound healing, as well as identifying and addressing any potential complications that may arise.

(8) (D) Checklists.

By using checklists, the nurse can ensure that all necessary steps are taken and that nothing is missed.

(9) (C) To confirm the correct patient, procedure and surgical site.

The time-out is a standardized procedure that is performed before the start of surgery to ensure that the correct patient, procedure and surgical site are confirmed by all members of the surgical team.

(10) (B) To increase communication and participation of patients in care decisions.

The goal of the Speak Up initiative is to increase communication and participation in care decisions by encouraging patients to ask questions, voice concerns and take an active role in preventing errors and ensuring their safety. While improving patient satisfaction, reducing health care costs and improving staff productivity may be beneficial, they are not the main objective of the initiative.

(11) (B) By ensuring all employees understand their roles and responsibilities in ensuring patient safety and holding them accountable for their actions.

High accountability is possible by ensuring all employees understand their roles and responsibilities in ensuring patient safety and holding them accountable for their actions. This way, everyone in the organization takes ownership of safety and is responsible for creating and maintaining a culture of safety.

(12) (A) It encourages staff to report errors without fear of retaliation.

The just-culture concept allows for open communication and learning from errors rather than punishing individuals for honest mistakes.

(13) (A) To improve the quality and safety of care.

Care bundles are a set of evidence-based practices that, when implemented together, have been shown to improve patient outcomes. They are designed to standardize care and reduce variation in practice, with the goal of improving the quality and safety of care.

(14) (C) To ensure that all necessary steps are taken before, during and after the procedure or treatment.

Checklists in a care bundle include specific steps that should be taken before, during and after the procedure or treatment. They are designed to standardize care and ensure that all necessary steps are taken to improve patient outcomes.

(15) (A) Elevating the head of the bed.

A checklist for preventing VAP might include elevating the head of the bed, oral care, stress ulcer prophylaxis and sedation vacation.

(16) (D) All of the above.

Algorithms used in care bundles typically include steps such as assessing the patient's pain level, identifying the cause of the pain, selecting an appropriate pain management technique, administering the chosen treatment, monitoring the patient's response to the treatment and adjusting the treatment as needed.

(17) (C) When new evidence emerges.

Algorithms used in care bundles are often reviewed and updated regularly to reflect changes in best practices and evidence-based care to provide optimal care to the patients.

(18) (A) To identify and evaluate potential hazards that could harm patients in a health care setting.

Patient safety assessment is the process of identifying and evaluating potential hazards that could harm patients in a health care setting and implementing measures to prevent these hazards.

(19) (D) Monitoring and evaluation.

The last step in the process of patient safety assessment is ongoing monitoring and evaluation of the effectiveness of interventions and making adjustments as necessary. This step is important to ensure that the implemented interventions are effective and to make any necessary adjustments to the process to continue to improve patient safety.

(20) (C) Identification of hazards.

The first step in conducting the patient safety assessment is identifying hazards, which in this case is medication errors. This involves reviewing patient data, monitoring incident reports and conducting on-site assessments to identify the root cause of the problem.

(21) (A) To identify problems and issues related to patient safety as soon as possible.

Patient safety reporting is the process of identifying and reporting incidents or conditions that have the potential to harm patients or negatively impact the quality of care provided. The goal is to identify problems and issues related to patient safety as soon as possible so that appropriate actions can be taken to prevent harm.

(22) (A) Incident reporting involves reporting incidents that have already caused harm, while near-miss reporting involves reporting incidents that have the potential to cause harm.

Incident reporting is an important tool for identifying problems that have already occurred, while near-miss reporting is a valuable tool for identifying potential problems that could occur in the future.

(23) (D) All of the above.

Root cause analysis is an important tool in patient safety reporting because it helps identify the underlying causes of incidents or adverse events, allows health care organizations to track and analyze data on incidents and near-misses and helps organizations identify ways to prevent incidents from happening again in the future. This allows health care organizations to take proactive measures to improve patient safety and prevent future incidents.

(24) (A) Root cause analysis, incident reporting, near-miss reporting, patient complaints.

By following these steps, the facility can identify the root cause of the problem, prevent future incidents and improve patient safety.

(25) (B) Document the suspected abuse in the patient's medical record.

The first step a nurse should take if they suspect a patient is a victim of abuse is to document the suspected abuse in the patient's medical record, including any observations or statements made by the patient. This documentation should be as detailed and specific as possible, including descriptions of any injuries or other observable evidence of abuse.

(26) (A) Reporting laws and regulations in the area.

It is important to remember that in many regions, health care providers are mandatory reporters, meaning that by law, they must report any suspicion of abuse to the authorities. Thus, the nurse should also be familiar with the reporting laws and regulations in the area and ensure compliance with them.

(27) (A) Assessing patients for SDOH during clinical encounters.

Providers can assess patients for SDOH during clinical encounters by using standardized screening tools or by asking specific questions related to a patient's living and working conditions, education or access to food or transportation.

(28) (A) Inform the supervisor or designated trafficking reporting contact.

This is the first step that should be taken, as it will trigger the proper protocols and procedures to report the case to the appropriate authorities, such as police or federal agencies dedicated to combating human trafficking.

(29) (C) Root Cause Analysis (RCA).

RCA is used to identify the symptoms, gather data, analyze the data and identify the root cause(s) of the problem. By identifying the root cause of a problem, RCA helps identify areas for improvement and develop strategies to prevent similar incidents from occurring in the future.

(30) (D) Failure Mode and Effects Analysis (FMEA).

By identifying potential failure modes and assessing their potential consequences, FMEA helps identify and prioritize potential risks and develop and implement control plans to mitigate them.

(31) (A) Safety rounds.

This method helps ensure that hazards and unsafe conditions are identified and addressed in a timely manner.

(32) (B) Safety huddles.

This method helps ensure that hazards and unsafe conditions are identified and addressed in a timely manner.

(33) (D) Risk assessment.

This helps ensure that patients receive safe and high-quality care and that adverse events are minimized.

(34) (C) Pick it up and dispose of it in the designated sharps container.

Any employee who notices a sharp object on the floor should be trained to pick it up and dispose of it in the designated sharps container.

(35) (C) To prevent the spread of organisms that can cause infection over long distances when suspended in the air.

Airborne precautions are implemented to reduce the risk of transmission from patients to health care providers and other patients. Airborne precautions are used when the organism can cause infection over long distances when suspended in the air, such as tuberculosis and rubeola.

(36) (C) Influenza and pertussis.

These pathogens are spread through droplets generated by talking, sneezing or coughing and can be easily transmitted through close contact with an infected person. Examples of such pathogens include influenza and pertussis.

(37) (A) To reduce the risk of transmission of pathogens that are acquired through direct or indirect contact, specifically MDROs.

Contact precautions are an essential measure in preventing the spread of pathogens that are acquired through direct or indirect contact, particularly MDROs such as MRSA and

VRE. These precautions are implemented to reduce the risk of transmission from patients to health care providers and other patients.

(38) (C) Using proper decontamination techniques, such as cleaning and disinfecting.

According to the CDC, one of the infection-control measures is to use proper decontamination. Techniques such as cleaning and disinfecting are used to prevent the spread of germs on frequently touched surfaces and medical equipment.

(39) (C) Implementing isolation protocols for patients with contagious illnesses.

According to the CDC, one of the infection-control measures is to implement isolation protocols for patients with contagious illnesses to prevent the spread of infection to other patients or health care workers.

(40) (C) Place the patient in a private room with a bathroom and limit the number of health care workers who enter the room.

According to the CDC, one of the measures to prevent the spread of infection is to implement isolation protocols for patients with contagious illnesses. This includes placing the patient in a private room with a bathroom and limiting the number of health care workers who enter the room. This will help prevent the spread of infection to other patients and health care workers.

(41) (D) Health care workers should perform hand hygiene with soap and water or an alcohol-based hand sanitizer before and after each patient contact.

According to WHO recommendations, proper strategies to prevent surgical site infections include proper hand hygiene, use of appropriate surgical attire, use of prophylactic antibiotics, proper wound management, proper patient positioning and proper environmental cleaning and disinfection.

(42) (C) Implementing infection-control measures, such as proper hand hygiene, use of PPE, appropriate cleaning and disinfection of health care environments and active surveillance for the presence of MDROs to identify and isolate infected individuals.

According to WHO recommendations, implementing infection-control measures is considered the most effective in preventing the spread of MDRO infections. Option A is not effective, as it delays the implementation of preventive measures. Option B is not effective, as it does not provide enough isolation and infection-control measures. And Option D is not effective as it may lead to the development and spread of MDROs.

(43) (C) To promote the appropriate use of antibiotics, including the use of narrow-spectrum antibiotics and the avoidance of unnecessary antibiotic use.

Antimicrobial stewardship programs aim to promote the appropriate use of antibiotics, including the use of narrow-spectrum antibiotics and the avoidance of unnecessary antibiotic use, in order to reduce the development and spread of MDROs.

(44) (D) Tracking the spread of antibiotic-resistant organisms using molecular epidemiology techniques.

Regular feedback and audits of antibiotic prescribing practices in an antimicrobial stewardship program can include tracking the spread of antibiotic-resistant organisms using molecular epidemiology techniques, such as whole genome sequencing and pulsed-field gel electrophoresis.

(45) (B) The ordering and preparing phase.

One of the most critical stages of the medication administration process is the transition point, which includes the ordering and preparing phase, where errors are more likely to occur.

(46) (C) They have a potential for significant harm when used in error.

Parenteral medications, including those administered via IV or subcutaneously, are considered high-alert medications due to the potential for significant harm when used in error.

(47) (D) All of the above.

Errors during medication administration can occur from a variety of sources, such as miscommunication between health care staff, incorrectly labeling or storing medications and lack of proper equipment or technology.

(48) (C) Implementing strict protocols for medication preparation and administration.

High-alert medications, such as parenteral medications, require special safeguards to minimize the risk of errors. One way to do this is by implementing strict protocols for medication preparation and administration, such as double-checking dosages and using barcode scanning technology.

(49) (C) During regular check-ups or follow-up appointments.

Patient medication education should be an ongoing process, not a one-time event. Health care providers should check in with patients regularly to ensure they understand and are following the medication regimen correctly. This can be done during regular check-ups or follow-up appointments.

(50) (C) The use of unnecessary or inappropriate medications.

Polypharmacy refers to the use of multiple medications or the use of potentially unnecessary or inappropriate medications. This can happen when a patient takes multiple medications to treat the same condition or when a medication does not match the diagnosis. It can also occur when a patient takes several medications that have similar actions to treat multiple conditions simultaneously or mix nutritional supplements or herbal products with medications.

(51) (B) The responsiveness of health care staff.

Patient satisfaction is a measure of patients' contentment with the health care services they receive and is influenced by various factors. The responsiveness of health care staff, the cleanliness and comfort of the facility, the effectiveness of treatment and the overall patient experience are just a few examples of factors that can affect patient satisfaction.

(52) (B) Surveys.

Surveys are the most commonly used method to gather feedback from patients regarding their satisfaction with health care services. These surveys may include questions about communication with providers, wait times and overall satisfaction with the care received.

(53) (A) To provide health care organizations with a benchmark for quality and safety of care.

These guidelines aim to ensure that health care organizations are providing the highest quality care to their patients and continuously striving to improve by measuring and evaluating patient satisfaction.

(54) (A) Administering standardized patient satisfaction surveys.

A standardized patient satisfaction survey should be validated and include questions about communication with providers, wait times and overall satisfaction with the care received. Regular administration of this survey allows health care organizations to gather feedback from patients and use it to identify areas for improvement.

(55) (D) To identify areas in need of improvement.

The goal of gathering feedback through standardized patient satisfaction surveys is to allow health care organizations to evaluate their performance and identify areas in need of improvement. This may include changes to the care provided, improving the patient experience or increasing staff.

(56) (C) By holding staff accountable for the care they provide.

The Joint Commission's guidelines recommend using patient satisfaction data in performance evaluations for individual providers and staff. By doing so, health care organizations can ensure that staff are held accountable for the care they provide and are motivated to improve patient satisfaction.

(57) (D) To increase confidence and reduce anxiety.

The main purpose of getting a second opinion for a patient is to increase confidence and reduce anxiety by providing a more informed decision about the patient's diagnosis and treatment options.

(58) (D) The patient's level of understanding and ability to participate in decision-making.

The most important piece of information for a nurse to know when referring a patient for a second opinion is the patient's level of understanding and ability to participate in decision-making. This information can help the specialist understand the patient's preferences and goals for treatment, as well as the support system available for the patient.

(59) (D) All of the above.

The nurse should gather all the information listed in the prompt. That includes Mary's medical history, current symptoms and concerns, current test results and imaging studies, previous treatment options, preferences and goals for treatment, insurance coverage and financial considerations, support system and availability of caregivers, cultural or linguistic considerations, level of understanding and ability to participate in decision-making and the availability and referral process for the specialist.

(60) (C) Identifying the problem that has occurred.

The first step in the service recovery process is identifying the problem that has occurred. This can be done through patient feedback or by monitoring and tracking incidents. It is important to accurately identify the problem in order to provide an appropriate resolution.

(61) (C) It shows the patient that the health care organization recognizes and takes responsibility for the problem.

A sincere apology can go a long way in mitigating the negative effects of a poor patient experience. It shows the patient that the health care organization recognizes and takes responsibility for the problem, which can help improve the patient's relationship with the health care organization and increase their satisfaction with the care they receive.

(62) (A) Complaints are minor issues related to room cleanliness, whereas grievances are serious issues related to patient care or Medicare billing.

Complaints are minor issues related to room cleanliness or food preferences. Grievances are issues regarding the patient's care, abuse or neglect, compliance with regulations or Medicare billing complaints.

(63) (D) Both the patient and the representative.

Both the patient and the representative can file a grievance, which is a formal or informal written or verbal complaint regarding the patient's care, abuse or neglect, compliance with regulations or Medicare billing complaints.

(64) (B) Decreased serum potassium levels.

In DKA, there is a relative insulin deficiency, leading to increased breakdown of fats and production of ketones. This process also results in the movement of potassium from the intracellular space to the extracellular space, leading to hypokalemia.

(65) (A) Loop diuretics.

Loop diuretics, such as furosemide, are commonly used in heart failure to reduce fluid overload and relieve symptoms of congestion by increasing urine output.

(66) (C) Obesity.

Obesity is a known risk factor for the development of DVT. Increased body weight can lead to venous stasis and impaired circulation, increasing the risk of blood clot formation.

(67) (D) Fever and chills.

Fever and chills are indicative of an inflammatory response and may suggest that the appendix has ruptured, leading to the spread of infection in the abdominal cavity.

(68) (B) Decreased oxygen saturation

Oxygen saturation reflects the amount of oxygen bound to hemoglobin in arterial blood. A decreased oxygen saturation indicates inadequate oxygenation and may require adjustments to the oxygen therapy to improve oxygen delivery to the patient.

(69) (B) Shortness of breath

While all of these symptoms could potentially indicate a problem, worsening heart failure would most likely present as increasing shortness of breath. This is due to fluid accumulation in the lungs, a result of the heart's inability to pump efficiently. The other symptoms may be seen in different conditions, but they are not typically associated with acute worsening heart failure.

(70) (C) Hyponatremia and hyperkalemia

Addison's disease, or primary adrenal insufficiency, results from insufficient production of adrenal hormones. This can lead to hyponatremia (low sodium levels) and hyperkalemia (high potassium levels) due to the lack of aldosterone, which helps regulate these electrolytes.

(71) (B) Pain management and NPO (nil per os/nothing by mouth)

Acute pancreatitis often presents with severe abdominal pain, which needs to be managed effectively. Keeping the patient NPO is crucial as it allows the pancreas to rest and recover. The other options may be necessary in different conditions, but they are not the primary focus in the management of acute pancreatitis.

(72) (C) Worsening or ascending paralysis

Guillain-Barré syndrome is a neurological disorder in which the body's immune system mistakenly attacks the nerves. Symptoms often start in the legs and progress upward. If the disease begins to affect the cranial nerves, which control speech and swallowing, it may indicate ascending paralysis, a serious condition that requires immediate medical intervention.

(73 (C) Oxygen therapy and anticoagulation as prescribed

In the case of a suspected pulmonary embolism, oxygen therapy can be used to address any hypoxia, while anticoagulation therapy can prevent further clot formation. While ambulation, diuretics, and chest physiotherapy may have roles in other respiratory conditions, they are not the priority in the management of PE.

(74) (B) Providing care that is sensitive to the cultural and linguistic needs of patients from diverse backgrounds.

Cultural competence is the ability of health care professionals to understand and respect the cultural backgrounds, beliefs and practices of patients and their families and to provide culturally appropriate care. Cultural sensitivity, which refers to the ability to recognize and respect cultural differences, is not enough.

(75) (B) Cultural humility.

Cultural humility involves being open and willing to learn about patients' cultural and linguistic backgrounds and striving to understand and appreciate their perspectives. This is crucial because it helps establish a strong therapeutic relationship with patients, which is essential for effective communication and care.

(76) (A) Call in a language specialist to interpret for the patient.

According to NCSBN guideline 3, "Language access: Nurses should be able to provide language assistance to patients and their families, either through the use of interpreters or through the use of translated materials." By calling in a language specialist, the nurse is ensuring that the patient's needs and symptoms are accurately communicated and addressed.

(77) (B) Sign languages.

Sign languages are used by individuals who are deaf or hard of hearing as a means of communication. They use a combination of hand gestures, facial expressions and body language to convey meaning. In this situation, sign language would be the most common way for the patient to communicate with health care providers.

(78) (C) Providing a variety of communication methods, including interpreter services and translated materials, to accommodate the cultural and linguistic needs of all patients.

Health care providers have a responsibility to ensure that all patients, regardless of their cultural and linguistic background, receive appropriate care. This includes providing a variety of communication methods, such as interpreter services and translated materials.

(79) (D) Interpreter services or translated materials in the preferred language.

Using interpreter services or translated materials in the preferred language is the most common solution for patients who speak a language other than the dominant language. This is because interpreter services or translated materials in the preferred language allow for effective communication between the patient and the health care provider.

(80) (D) D-dimer blood test

The D-dimer blood test is commonly used as a screening tool to detect the presence of a blood clot. If the D-dimer level is elevated, further imaging tests, such as a CT pulmonary angiogram, may be performed to confirm the diagnosis of pulmonary embolism.

(81) (B) pH 7.32, PaCO2 48 mmHg, HCO3- 22 mEq/L

Metabolic acidosis is characterized by a low pH (<7.35) and a decreased bicarbonate (HCO3-) level (<22 mEq/L). The compensatory response includes an increased respiratory rate to eliminate excess carbon dioxide (PaCO2 >45 mmHg).

(82) (D) By inhibiting gastric acid secretion

Explanation: Proton pump inhibitors (PPIs) work by irreversibly blocking the gastric H+/K+ ATPase pump, which is responsible for the final step of gastric acid secretion. This reduces acid production in the stomach, providing relief and promoting healing of peptic ulcers.

(83 (C) Deep vein thrombosis (DVT)

Prolonged immobility increases the risk of developing deep vein thrombosis (DVT) due to reduced blood flow, venous stasis, and endothelial damage. Patients should be assessed for DVT risk and preventive measures, such as early ambulation and prophylactic anticoagulation, should be implemented.

(84) (B) Unconscious attitudes or stereotypes toward certain groups of people.

Implicit bias refers to the unconscious attitudes or stereotypes toward certain groups of people that can influence perceptions, attitudes and behaviors. It is different from attitudes and beliefs that people are aware of and can control.

(85) (B) Disparities in the quality of care that patients receive.

Implicit bias can lead to disparities in the quality of care that patients receive in health care. For example, it can lead to a lack of trust and communication between the health care provider and the patient, which can result in lower-quality care.

(86) (C) Implementing policies and procedures to promote diversity, equity and inclusion.

Health care organizations can play a role in reducing the effects of implicit bias by implementing policies and procedures to promote diversity, equity and inclusion.

(87) (D) Receive training on cultural competence and awareness of their own biases.

To reduce the effects of implicit bias, it is important for health care providers to receive training on cultural competence and awareness of their own biases.

(88) (B) Educating patients and families about healthy behaviors.

One of the key responsibilities of a nurse in health maintenance is educating patients and families about healthy behaviors, such as regular exercise, good nutrition and adequate sleep and how they can implement these behaviors in their daily lives.

(89) (C) Implement infection-control measures.

One of the steps that a nurse can take is implementing infection-control measures, such as hand hygiene and the use of PPE, to prevent the spread of infectious diseases in health care settings.

(90) (D) Provide education and resources to patients and families.

One way a nurse can encourage patient self-management and self-care is by providing education and resources to patients and families to take an active role in their health.

(91) (C) Assess and address the patient's health status, screen for common diseases and refer for follow-up care.

In the case of a patient with heart disease, the nurse's role is crucial in ensuring the patient's health maintenance. This includes assessing the patient's health status, identifying risk factors and developing a care plan to address them. It also involves screening for common diseases, such as heart disease, and referring the patient for appropriate follow-up care if necessary.

(92) (B) Proper nutrition and early disease detection.

The ANA (American Nurses Association) encourages nurses to educate patients and the public about various health topics. However, one of the primary areas of focus is promoting proper nutrition and early disease detection. Nurses play a vital role in educating individuals about the importance of maintaining a healthy diet, making informed food choices, and understanding the impact of nutrition on overall health.

Additionally, nurses also emphasize the significance of early disease detection through regular screenings and check-ups, empowering individuals to take proactive steps in managing their health and preventing the progression of diseases.

(93) (C) Vaccination.

The ANA supports the use of vaccines as a safe and effective way to prevent the spread of infectious diseases and encourages nurses to educate patients about the importance of vaccination.

(94) (A) Access to affordable health care, healthy food options and safe housing.

The ANA encourages nurses to advocate for policies that support health maintenance and disease prevention, such as access to affordable health care, healthy food options and safe housing.

(95) (B) Decreased blood pressure

ACE inhibitors act by inhibiting the conversion of angiotensin I to angiotensin II, a potent vasoconstrictor. This results in vasodilation, decreased systemic vascular resistance, and lower blood pressure.

(96) (C) Health literacy is a necessary condition for making informed decisions about one's health.

As defined by the WHO, health literacy is an individual's ability to comprehend, interpret and act on health information in order to make informed decisions and take appropriate actions to maintain and improve their health.

(97) (D) All of the above.

Nurses should assess the patient's health literacy level, communicate by using clear and simple language and provide written materials that are easy to read and understand. They should also encourage patients to participate in their care and ask questions.

(98) (C) Use clear, simple language and provide written materials that are easy to read and understand.

Health literacy is important for nurses to consider when interacting with patients. They should assess the patient's health literacy level; communicate in clear, simple language; and provide written materials that are easy to read and understand.

(99) (C) Provide the patient with balanced and accurate information about the benefits and risks of vaccines.

The ANA supports the use of vaccines as a safe and effective way to prevent the spread of infectious diseases and encourages nurses to educate patients about the importance of vaccination.

(100) (C) The continuous assessment and adaptation of teaching strategies.

The patient education process is dynamic and continuous, requiring health care professionals to continuously assess and evaluate the patient's understanding and progress. This allows for a personalized and effective educational experience and ensures that patients are empowered to take an active role in their own health and well-being.

(101) (C) To recognize the patient as a unique individual.

Individualized care in nursing recognizes that each patient is unique and has specific experiences, behaviors, feelings and perceptions, including the events associated with their illness, home life, work, physical indicators and preferred coping strategies. The main goal of this approach is to provide care that is tailored to the patient's individual needs and circumstances, rather than applying a generic treatment plan to all patients.

(102) (A) Wearing gloves during patient care

Standard precautions are the basic infection prevention practices that apply to all patient care, regardless of the suspected or confirmed infection status. Wearing gloves during patient care is a standard precaution as it helps to prevent the transmission of microorganisms from both patients and healthcare workers.

(103) (C) A group of health care professionals with different areas of expertise working together.

In this case, an interdisciplinary approach to care is likely to be the most effective in meeting the patient's needs. This approach brings together different health care professionals with different areas of expertise to work together in a coordinated manner, pooling their knowledge and skills to provide comprehensive, holistic care that addresses the patient's physical, emotional and social needs.

(104) (C) Schedule regular times for the nurse and physician team to meet and discuss the patient's care.

Regular meetings can help promote open and direct communication between the nurse and physician team and prevent misunderstandings that can negatively impact patient care. Ignoring communication issues, encouraging competition or promoting a hierarchical approach can hinder collaboration and negatively impact patient care.

(105) (D) All of the above.

The practice of interprofessional rounding brings together physicians, nurses, social workers and other members of the health care team to discuss patient care and treatment plans.

(106) (C) Physicians, nurses, social workers and other members of the health care team.

Interprofessional rounding involves a team approach to patient care, where different health care professionals participate in regular meetings to discuss patient conditions and treatment plans. This typically includes physicians, nurses, social workers and other members of the health care team who are involved in the patient's care.

(107) (B) Consult with the patient's primary physician to make adjustments to the medication regimen.

In the case of adverse effects from a patient's medication regimen, the interprofessional team should consult with the patient's primary physician to make adjustments to the medication regimen. Interprofessional rounding provides a platform for the health care team to share information and coordinate care, which includes addressing any potential issues, such as adverse effects from medication.

(108) (D) The entire health care team, including the patient and the family.

Updating a patient's care plan during interprofessional rounding is a collaborative effort involving the entire health care team. The patient's primary physician may have the ultimate responsibility for making decisions about the patient's treatment, but the care plan should reflect input from all members of the health care team, including the nurse responsible for the patient's care, as well as the patient and their family.

(109) (C) Daily or weekly.

The frequency of interprofessional rounding in a health care facility can vary. Some facilities hold daily rounds, while others hold weekly team meetings or other regular opportunities for communication. The specific frequency is based on the needs of the patients and the health care facility and may change over time as patient needs and the health care system evolve.

(110) (C) By leading to confusion, frustration and a lack of trust in the health care system.

The lack of understanding by patients can negatively impact the health care system, as it can lead to confusion, frustration and a lack of trust in the health care system. Patients may not understand why they are being referred, how to schedule appointments or what steps to take after visiting a specialist, which can negatively impact their overall experience with the health care system.

(111) (A) Identifying and assigning roles and responsibilities among health care providers.

A specific action to achieve coordinated care in primary care practices is identifying and assigning roles and responsibilities among health care providers. This helps promote open communication, facilitate smooth transitions of care and ensure that patients receive high-quality, high-value health care.

(112) (B) Managing medications.

A broad care coordination approach in primary care practices is medication management. It is one of several approaches—including teamwork among health care providers, care management programs, health information technology and the patient-centered medical home model—that aim to improve health care delivery and ensure that patients receive high-quality, high-value health care.

(113) (A) Facilitating smooth transitions of care.

Facilitating smooth transitions of care involves ensuring a seamless transfer of information and responsibility between health care providers, promoting open communication and ensuring that patients receive high-quality, high-value health care.

(114) (A) Health information technology.

A broad care coordination approach in primary care practices is health information technology. For example, using an electronic health record system can help health care providers share information and track a patient's care, leading to better coordination and improved health care delivery.

(115) (C) To develop solutions to address patient care issues.

The main goal of collaborative problem-solving in health care is to develop solutions to address patient care issues. For example, a team of nurses, doctors and pharmacy staff might come together to identify the root causes of medication errors and implement solutions to address the issue.

(116) (B) Implementing a standardized communication protocol.

An example of a task performed during collaborative problem-solving in health care is implementing a standardized communication protocol. For example, a team of health care professionals might identify poor communication between providers as a root cause of medication errors and implement a standardized communication protocol to address the issue and improve patient care.

(117) (C) Public health departments.

Public health departments are a type of resource available in the community that can provide information on public health issues and outbreaks, as well as patient education and vaccination programs. For example, nurses working in community settings may need to be familiar with public health departments in order to stay informed about outbreaks and access resources for patient education.

(118) (C) To provide primary care and other health services, such as vaccinations and screenings, to people in the community.

Community health clinics provide primary care and other health services, such as vaccinations and screenings, to people in the community, regardless of their ability to pay. These clinics serve an important role in improving access to health care for underserved populations and can play a critical role in promoting public health.

(119) (C) The patient is at risk of harm to self due to confusion or agitation

Restraints should only be used as a last resort, when all other alternatives to ensure safety have been exhausted, and the patient poses a significant risk of harm to themselves or others. Non-compliance, frequent requests for assistance, or refusal to eat are not appropriate reasons for the use of restraints.

(120) (C) Every 2 hours

The nurse should check on a restrained patient's circulation, mobility, and comfort at least every 2 hours. This is to ensure that the restraints are not causing harm, such as impaired circulation, skin damage, or unnecessary discomfort. Additionally, during each check, the nurse should also reassess the need for continued use of restraints.

(121) (C) Immediately remove the IV catheter

Infiltration occurs when IV fluid or medications leak into the surrounding tissue. Symptoms may include swelling, discomfort, or coolness around the IV site. If infiltration is suspected, the first action should be to stop the infusion and remove the

IV catheter to prevent further damage. Warm or cold compresses may be used afterward depending on the type of solution that has infiltrated.

(122) (C) A vein that is straight and feels bouncy when palpated

A straight vein that feels bouncy when palpated is the most desirable for IV insertion. These characteristics often indicate a healthy, full vein that will allow for a smooth IV catheter insertion. While large, visible, or superficial veins might seem appealing, they are not necessarily the best choice. They could be fragile or tortuous which can make the insertion more difficult and increase the risk for complications. Using a vein in the non-dominant arm is a good consideration for patient comfort, but it's not the most important factor when choosing an appropriate vein for IV insertion.

(123) (B) To help Mr. Smith regain or maintain his mobility.

The goal is to help him regain or maintain his mobility. The nurse will consider Mr. Smith's ability to move and perform basic functional tasks and any physical limitations or conditions, such as muscle weakness or joint pain, and develop a plan that may include physical therapy, exercises and the use of assistive devices.

(124) (B) To assess a patient's risk of falling.

The TUG test measures a patient's ability to stand up from a seated position, walk a short distance and return to a seated position. It is commonly used by medical professionals to assess a patient's risk of falling, as it provides an indication of mobility and balance.

(125) (B) A patient's balance, stability and ability to perform functional activities.

The BBS test measures a patient's balance, stability and ability to perform functional activities, such as reaching, turning and stepping. This test provides an indication of a patient's mobility and overall functional ability.

(126) (A) To measure a patient's ability to perform basic activities of daily living.

The Barthel Index of Activities of Daily Living is a test used to measure a patient's ability to perform basic activities of daily living, such as bathing, dressing and toileting. This test provides an overall assessment of a patient's functional ability and independence.

(127) (B) The FTSST test.

The FTSST test measures a patient's ability to stand up from a seated position and sit back down again. This test provides an assessment of a patient's lower body strength and muscle function. It is commonly used by medical professionals to evaluate a patient's overall mobility and functional ability.

(128) (B) To measure a patient's ability to reach forward while maintaining balance.

The Functional Reach Test measures a patient's ability to reach forward while maintaining balance. This test provides an assessment of a patient's stability and balance. It is commonly used by medical professionals to evaluate a patient's overall mobility and functional ability.

(129) (D) The Barthel Index of Activities of Daily Living.

The Barthel Index of Activities of Daily Living measures a patient's ability to perform basic activities of daily living, such as bathing, dressing and toileting.

(130) (A) The TUG test.

A medical professional would use the TUG test to assess a patient's risk of falling.

(131) (C) The BBS test.

The BBS measures a patient's balance, stability and ability to perform functional activities, such as reaching, turning and stepping.

(132) (B) The FTSST test.

After a knee replacement surgery, a medical professional would use the FTSST test to assess a patient's lower body strength and muscle function.

(133) (A) The TUG test.

A medical professional would use the TUG test to assess a patient's risk of falling.

(134) (D) The Barthel Index of Activities of Daily Living.

A medical professional would use the Barthel Index of Activities of Daily Living to assess a patient's ability to perform basic activities of daily living, such as bathing, dressing and toileting.

(135) (C) The BBS test.

A medical professional would use the BBS to assess a patient's balance, stability and ability to perform functional activities, such as reaching, turning and stepping.

(136) (D) Patient is able to move with minimal assistance.

The FMS is a commonly used scale to grade mobility on a scale of 0 to 4, with 0 indicating that the patient is unable to move and requires full assistance and 4 indicating that the patient is able to move independently. A grade of 3 on the FMS indicates that the patient is able to move with minimal assistance.

(137) (B) Patient is able to move but requires significant assistance.

A grade of 1 indicates that the patient is able to move but requires significant assistance.

(138) (C) Patient is able to move but requires moderate assistance.

A grade of 2 indicates that the patient is able to move but requires some assistance to do so.

(139) (D) Patient is able to move independently.

A grade of 4 indicates that the patient is able to move and perform activities of daily living independently, without any assistance or with only minimal help.

(140) (A) Patient is unable to move and requires full assistance.

A patient with a grade of 0 is unable to move and requires full assistance, meaning the person is unable to perform movements on their own and requires support from others for all mobility tasks.

(141) (A) 0.

Patients who have recently had a stroke and are unable to stand or walk without assistance are likely to have a grade of 0 on the FMS, indicating that they are unable to move and require full assistance from others for all mobility tasks.

(142) (C) 2.

A patient who has recently recovered from a broken leg and has been doing physical therapy to regain mobility is likely to have a grade of 2 on the FMS, indicating that they are able to move but require moderate assistance with some tasks, such as standing or walking for a long distance. This level of mobility may improve with additional physical therapy and rehabilitation.

(143) (C) 2.

The patient described in the question is likely to be assigned a grade of 2. This grade indicates that the patient is able to move but requires moderate assistance, such as someone to be with them for safety.

(144) (A) 0.

Patients who have been bedridden for several months due to a serious illness are likely to have a grade of "0" on the FMS.

(145) (C) To provide comprehensive evaluation and develop a treatment plan.

The main goal of physical therapy in the case of a patient who has recently had hip replacement surgery is to provide a comprehensive evaluation of the patient's current level of mobility, strength, flexibility and function and then develop an individualized treatment plan to help the patient regain mobility.

(146) (C) Three times a week.

Physical therapy sessions would typically be scheduled for the patient three times a week until their goals are met, and the person is able to move around independently.

(147) (D) All of the above.

When conducting a health history assessment, nurses typically gather information from multiple sources. This includes talking with patients about their medical history, current symptoms and medications, reviewing medical records and laboratory results and asking family members or caregivers for additional information.

(148) (C) Ask the patient about medical history and current symptoms.

The first step that a nurse typically takes when conducting a health history assessment is talking with patients and asking about their medical history, current symptoms and any medications or supplements they are taking. This information can help the nurse identify any risk factors or underlying conditions that may impact patients' care.

(149) (B) Before the day of discharge, notify the patient and the designated family or caregivers of the anticipated discharge date and time.

This step is crucial, as it helps the patient and the family or designated caregivers prepare for the patient's discharge and ensure that they are ready for any post-discharge care that may be necessary.

(150) (D) To promote compliance and prevent any improper administration of medications.

The comprehensive medication list should include the name, dosage, frequency and any potential side effects or interactions of the patient's medications. Reviewing this list with the patient and the family or designated caregivers ensures that the medication schedule aligns with the patient's daily routine and lifestyle to promote compliance and prevent any improper administration.